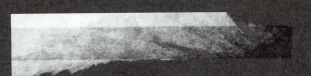

LIFE'S BLOOD

Madeline Marget

SIMON & SCHUSTER

New York   London   Toronto   Sydney   Tokyo   Singapore

SIMON & SCHUSTER
Simon & Schuster Building
Rockefeller Center
1230 Avenue of the Americas
New York, New York 10020

Designed by Carla Weise/Levavi & Levavi
Manufactured in the United States of America

10 9 8 7 6 5 4 3 2 1

Library of Congress Cataloging-in-Publication Data

Marget, Madeline.
Life's blood / Madeline Marget.
p.   cm.
Includes bibliographical references and index.
1. Leukemia—Popular works. 2. Bone marrow—Transplantation.
3. Bone marrow—Transplantation—Patients. 4. Rappeport, Joel.
I. Title.
RC643.M34   1992
616.1′5—dc20   91-47534
CIP
ISBN 0-671-69488-X

Contents

When fainting Nature called for aid,
  And hovering Death prepared the blow,
His vigorous remedy displayed
  The power of art without the show.

—Samuel Johnson,
    "On the Death of Dr. Robert Levet"

Introduction

I first met the hematologist Joel Rappeport in 1986, after my sister developed acute megakaryocytic leukemia, a particularly rare and deadly form of the disease. Her treatment was to be a bone marrow transplant, and I was the donor. On a dismal November morning Roberta was admitted to the hospital, and I sloshed through a dirty, premature snow to the hematology outpatient clinic, where I had an appointment for a checkup with Rappeport. I was furious and sad, filled with dread. I didn't like doctors, I didn't like hospitals, and I knew all about high-tech medicine and its practitioners. I knew they were cold and arrogant, but I knew that when you were sick enough to need them you had no choice but to put up with them. I was trapped.

A couple of weeks earlier, when I had talked to Rappeport on the phone, he'd snarled at me. Roberta had just left his office upset and angry. She'd found him cold. She'd quoted Rappeport as saying that the massive doses of radiation and chemotherapeutic drugs she'd receive would "really beat her up," and that she had only a 15 percent chance of survival. I'd called Rappeport in disbelief. How could it be that we were about to take such extreme measures when the likelihood of success was so low? He'd almost hung up on me. He said he wished "you people"—my sister and I—would leave him alone, to get on with it.

Before my actual meeting with Rappeport, I sat in the waiting room for two hours. A couple of men talked about a third who hadn't "fought it" as hard as they thought they were. A young doctor talked on the phone, repeatedly explaining to a patient that she couldn't treat her without seeing her. Everything seemed to move slowly, people seemed to be taking their time. Finally, a man came and said my name. I jumped up and took the hand he offered me. I knew who he was, but I didn't admit it. He hadn't introduced himself, and I was eager to put a doctor in his place. "Who are you?" I said. He looked surprised at my question, but he answered.

I had heard that Joel Rappeport was a genius. I understood that the work he did was highly specialized and that many—I then thought most—of his patients died. I could not see why anyone would want to be a hematologist, and I expected him to be a very peculiar man, a strange person absorbed in arcane detail. As soon as I saw him, I knew that I was wrong. He looked tired, and kind. He smiled at me and shifted his body as if he were unsure of himself.

In the examining room, though, his touch was gentle, and he was precise and knowledgeable as he explained the purpose and risks of bone marrow donation. Then he leaned against the window frame, looked outside at the dreary weather, and talked. I had denied the grief I felt pressing on me. This—giving my bone marrow—was just something I had to do, I'd said. A thing any decent person would do. But Rappeport referred, casually and without inflection, to "all you're going through," and he did not hide his own sadness. His evident feeling, along with his complete lack of affectation or veneer, showed his intimacy with his great and frightening subject. I was moved and comforted.

I asked him what the greatest danger to Roberta was, if she survived the transplant itself. "Oh," he said, a shrug in his voice, "the leukemia coming back." I was shocked at his casual use of the word "leukemia," one of the most horrifying I knew. Leukemia existed and was likely to kill. And yet he, with a worldwide reputation and time to talk, had chosen to tangle with it. And so I did not believe my sister would die. I forgave the long, unexplained wait I'd put in that morning, and I dismissed the inadequacies of the lackadaisical nurse who'd been unable to find a vein—accessible to every other technician I'd ever encountered—from which to draw a blood sample. I put aside Rappeport's previous response to Roberta and to me. Instead, I concentrated on the hope his sincerity and knowledge offered.

Over time, I watched him in the clinic and at the bedside, listened to him in lecture halls and private conversations, and learned from his colleagues and other doctors and scientists and—most of all, by far—from his patients. Through them, I came to understand and feel the difficult reality of the hope he offers.

Rappeport is a burdened, troubled man. For over twenty-five years his world has been filled with pain and fright. His bone marrow transplant patients are young people afflicted with fatal diseases. It is sad and terrible to see their plight, and inspiring to see their bravery. Rappeport, cranky and difficult, has been devoted to his patients all his professional life. Because of his dedication and the time in which he lives, he has increasingly been able to save them.

Hematology is at the very center of today's explosion of biological knowledge. The first experiments in altering human genes in order to cure devastating illness are taking place today, using blood cells. The study of blood is integral to immunology, too. And because blood is not only terribly complicated but also highly accessible, it allows ongoing, repeated examination. It can be drawn, over and over again, from the same person, so that the course of many diseases can be described and then understood, and finally the conditions themselves can be cured.

Bone marrow produces blood. A bone marrow transplant is an extreme and dangerous way of curing many illnesses—not only leukemia and other malignancies but also hereditary diseases. It is *not* a magic bullet, but it often works, and it does so when nothing else will. Roberta would have been dead within weeks of my initial meeting with Rappeport had she not gone ahead with the transplant. Nearly all the other patients I describe in the chapters that follow had no alternative to a transplant either, except premature death, and many of them are now well.

In addition to the individual cures, important and urgent as each of them is, there is the knowledge gained from them. Because blood is pervasive and bone marrow basic, a transplant offers the opportunity to track cells, to study their normal as well as abnormal development and function. It's a chance—a repeated, continuous chance, presented through many patients, over decades—to get to the fundamental causes of disease. Hematology is an intellectually stimulating science as well as a desperately needed medical specialty. Hematopoiesis—the formation and development of blood cells—is a microcosm of all physical human development. A very good doctor who specializes in bone marrow transplants combines individual cure with scientific discovery; his patient is both his charge and his laboratory.

When I asked Rappeport what his greatest wish for the future was, he was startled by the question, but said, anyway, what he clearly regards as obvious. He wants eradication of the terrible diseases his patients suffer. He knows that this will come through science, especially through the new biological tools and understanding of molecular genetics. That makes hope realistic, because with these means, cure has been accomplished and is in the making. Rappeport watches his patients vomit, he sees their hair fall out, he sees them get sicker than they were when they started—sometimes lastingly so. Often, he sees them die. He blames himself when things go wrong. And yet he knows, with each person, that he may be able to help. Rappeport is both intensely tenacious and notably insecure. His personality matches his moment in scientific and medical history.

Nevertheless, giving a lecture to medical students, he seems absolutely sure of himself and unequivocally positive about hematology. His talk seems spontaneous but is extremely well rehearsed. He's given this speech, with variations and updates, for years. Rappeport, now professor of medicine at Yale as well as head of the bone marrow transplant program there, knows just what he's doing; he's highly conscious of his responsibility as a teacher. James Watson, whose passionate personality and discovery—with Francis Crick—of DNA qualify him as the ultimate twentieth-century scientist, says young people today choose banking or law in preference to science not because they're greedy for money but because science is so *hard*. There are so many *facts* now, he says. So what you have to do is tell them they don't have to know so many facts, because the truth is that no one person can assimilate all of them.[1]

Rappeport, too, is careful not to scare students off, and he succeeds in making hematology sound fascinating, appealing rather than daunting. Speaking in a medical school amphitheater to a crowd of future doctors, he makes the promise of his work, especially of bone marrow transplants, limitless. They'll hear other specialties are central, but they're not. *Hematopoiesis* is central.

Everybody laughs, including Rappeport. He shows slides of normal and abnormal cells, and sick patients made well. Two pictures reproduce a Scott's Turfbuilder ad. First, in front of a suburban ranch house, there's barren soil. The blades of grass that are Rappeport's metaphor for blood's developing cells are absent. This is nonfunctioning bone marrow. That's the way it is, he says, before a transplant. Then the slide projector clicks and the thickest of green lawns appears: stem cells have engrafted. And as a result, red cells are again nourishing the body, multiple forms of white cells are protecting it against infection's invasions, and platelets are effectively at work preventing hemorrhage.

Every single time he gives this talk Rappeport acts surprised—full of wonder—at the victory he's announcing. Rappeport, no phony, is nevertheless an actor. His delight may be feigned, but it is purposeful. He wants his audience to find his information exciting news, so that the best students will work with him, in hematology, toward cure. And so he does not talk, in this initial, proselytizing lecture, about the darkness with which he lives. Instead, he makes it seem that nothing could be more fun than the life of a hematologist, especially one who does bone marrow transplants.

Brian Smith, a hematologist especially interested in immunology, is Rappeport's closest colleague and very good friend. He trained under Rappeport over fifteen years ago and says, "Joel was the one who, when you had a question, was *always* there." He also says, shaking his head, "Want to maintain a professional relationship, with distance? Joel won't let you." But Smith followed Rappeport from Boston—where Rappeport worked until the end of 1987—to New Haven. At Yale, Smith is associate professor of laboratory medicine, internal medicine, and pediatrics, and is also director of research for the bone marrow transplant unit. "Czar of all the Russias," Smith jokes, as he sits in his small office across the hall from the large research laboratory he heads, and near the clinical immunology laboratory he also directs.

Rappeport says all his investigative work is collaborative. Smith says, "In addition to those projects where Joel's been the primary person, there are all those that, if he were not there having the interest and enthusiasm for participating in things at the bench level, at the clinical level, at a variety of levels, would just never have happened."

Brian Smith says that technology drives science; the right technique for staining cells under the microscope, for example, leads to the identification of a property or entity previously unknown, and that in turn defines critical questions. Rappeport, as if stating the obvious, points out that science always comes first, that engendering ideas and formulating problems is the hard, slow part, after which technology is relatively fast and easy.

Smith can mimic a patient's mannerisms without mockery, and he has a gift for offering a simple explanation of difficult science without diminishing or omitting his subject's complexity, variety, and uncertainties. For example, all *cytogenetics* means, he says, is looking at chromosomes under the microscope in order to differentiate the normal from the abnormal.

Rappeport says good research and good patient care "aren't mutually exclusive. It just takes longer, that's all. It makes the day longer."

"The worst time in a hospital," says one of Rappeport's former patients, "is the weekends, when the action stops. Joel is there at three in the morning. Sunday, Monday, all the time. Like the Marx Brothers, with a cookie in one hand and coffee in the other."

Rappeport says that, when he started, he didn't realize how physically punishing he'd find his work as he aged. He's still at the hospital until midnight, but in middle age he admits to exhaustion, complains—at length, repeatedly, and with a touch of hysteria in his voice—about the demands he nonetheless does not delegate or refuse: calls from patients, teaching duties, the rounds and committee assignments he refers to as "good citizenship," and above all the daily patient care.

"If Joel put boundaries," says Smith, "that he'd always be home by seven, that he'd limit his practice to X number of patients, then he'd be operating at less than the 100 to 120 percent speed that's satisfactory to him." Smith believes that most doctors are motivated by a desire to do good, but says, in reflecting upon Rappeport's dedication to his field, "Joel's like 10 percent, 15 percent, 20 percent of doctors, depending upon one's optimism on any particular day."

Chronic myelogenous leukemia—often referred to as CML—is a form of leukemia especially intriguing to researchers, partly because it's known to originate in the stem cell—that is, at the very beginning of blood cell division. When hematologists talk about CML in the abstract, they focus on the insight into biology they may gain from building on what they know. But CML is also a disease that fatally afflicts many people. In Yale's hematology outpatient clinic, a fifty-five-year-old woman sits, legs swinging, on an examining table as Rappeport spends an hour and a half telling her what she already knows. She is a bright person who has learned about her condition; she is in the clinic to see Rappeport for a second opinion. Her husband sits with his hands shaking over a tape recorder. He and his wife find this a useful device when they go to the doctor because, she explains, they get nervous and forget exactly what has been said.

A young doctor who is also in the examining room doesn't like the tape recorder. He shakes his head and raises his eyebrows. He says the woman, whom he glimpsed in the waiting room, is the type who makes trouble for doctors. Before going into the examining room he adds a gratuitous insult, saying that because "she is obese," it would be impossible to feel her spleen. Rappeport has no trouble finding it. The patient is plump, not obese; a healthy-looking, if pale, middle-aged woman. There is no indication she intends to "make trouble." The only evident hostility is the young doctor's. The patient's husband looks like an old sailor, wearing a jersey with wide blue and white horizontal stripes and with a white beard that runs from sideburn to sideburn circling the lower half of his face. In fact, he works with computers.

The genetic change that exists in chronic myelogenous leukemia has been precisely identified. In CML a piece of chromosome 22 changes places with a fragment of chromosome 9. The result, called the Philadelphia Chromosome, is a visible change in the afflicted person's DNA, one that differentiates this form of the disease from other leukemias. The aberration occurs only in the bone marrow cells, and only in some of those. It doesn't happen anywhere else in the body—not, for example, in liver cells or skin cells or ovum cells or sperm cells. Though it involves the genes, it's not hereditary; the affected person is not born with this alteration. So far, knowing about the Philadelphia Chromosome hasn't improved the treatment of people sick with leukemia, but like other genetic knowledge, chromosomal identification of CML offers hope of the kind Watson says doctors want: If you know precisely where a disease is, you can find out more about it and then somehow excise it and only it, sparing the person.[2]

Rappeport's patient wants to make sure she understands her disease and its probable course. She does. Once it goes into a blast crisis—the accelerated stage, when malformed and misfunctioning white cells take over—there will be no way to save her. If she were younger, a bone marrow transplant might cure the disease,[3] but in her case there is no cure. The crisis could develop in two months or might not come for twenty years. In the meantime, there are drugs with few side effects she should take. They might help. And she can live as she wishes; no activity will be more harmful to her now than it was before she got sick. Nor will any activity in which she engages enhance her odds at a long life. Her husband indicates that he cannot accept this last information. What about diet? What about positive thinking? What about a doctor he's read of in the papers, heard of on the radio, mentioned by a friend? Rappeport, involved and attentive, considers every question but replies, positively and point by point, that there are no miracles.

In the hospital, as Rappeport makes rounds, the mother of a twenty-year-old, dying in the intensive care unit, asks a question. Her daughter had had a bone marrow transplant a year earlier; now the disease has returned, and she has pneumonia as well. She cannot speak; a tube, attached to a respirator, goes down her throat. She is emaciated and bald. Her skin has a yellowish tinge because her liver is failing. The mother asks about graft-versus-host disease—sometimes a lethal problem but often a treatable one. Rappeport discusses the mother's question with energy; he has walked quickly back down the hall to talk to her.

Always, in the hospitals and clinics where catastrophic illness predominates, there is the endless waiting for the doctor to come, for the answer to be certain. In hematology, uncertainty—one of the hardest emotions to confront—still prevails. The patient doesn't know when there will be a crisis or—if the treatment is intense and extensive—what the long-term effects will be. The doctor doesn't know, either.

"We will *all* die," Joel Rappeport says, but he uses these words as a statement of denial—it prefaces or concludes or brackets talk of how he's going to try to prevent a particular person from dying *then*. He says it with—almost—a smile; it's a reminder that none of us is different from the one in peril. In his practice, with its emphasis on radical treatment—bone marrow transplantation—the patients are usually children and adolescents, and people in their twenties and thirties.

Why be a hematologist, or learn about one? Why get close to people likely to die, why submit yourself to watching them suffer? Or worse, turn away from them when they are? Somebody has to do it, Rappeport says. And things are improving. And then, there's just the question of finding a job that fits his own impatient, driven nature. "I couldn't have been a dermatologist," says Rappeport. "I wouldn't have been good with a neurotic itch. I don't think anybody thinks I'd be good at that." He talks about going to patients' funerals, about the responsibility he feels toward their families afterward. And when his patients do live, he says, "I get some vicarious gain out of it, too." He shifts his body in his seat, trying to make himself clearer. "You've taken whatever it is—the Fates—and slapped them in the face."

The day he says this, Rappeport's in a combative mood, but it isn't that side of him that draws people close, or that explains his importance and that of his work. What does attract others, and what matters about him, is the knowledge and intensity with which he helps sick, scared people who—right this minute—are suffering from diseases that would have killed them, for sure, in midcentury. He helps them with means that didn't exist then and that probably won't be needed in another decade—or maybe two or three. Although we hate to think it, his kind of medicine is relevant to all of us. It could be any of us with leukemia or lymphoma or aplastic anemia or any of a huge number of potentially fatal acquired and genetic diseases, sitting in a doctor's office or a clinic, lying in a hospital bed. The newest science and medicine could save us now, and is likely to in the future.

The father of a patient says that Rappeport looks like a beagle. It's a fond description, and true. He also always has bags under his eyes and habitually needs a haircut. His tie is loose and its knot perpetually askew. Pictures of him as a young man show a self-assured, even cocky, football player. In his fifties now, he's physically smaller than he was then; his clothes hang on him, and he's slightly bent. He walks with his body pitched forward. His face in repose (which it usually isn't) is stern. When a patient calls with a problem that alarms him, his voice stays matter-of-fact and authoritative, but his complexion turns a purplish gray.

His worry is the product of a quarter century of heartbreaking effort, but his dissatisfaction is that of a perfectionist who doesn't quite have it yet. Still, whether or not there are miracles is a matter of definition. Rappeport knows there's been progress, and he's sure there'll be more. The reality of that sometimes stumbling, sometimes exhilarating, always critically serious progress is the subject of this book.

ONE

Fundamentals

*B*one marrow, the body's blood producer, is its third largest organ, after the skin and the liver. It is extraordinarily sensitive to a variety of toxins and drugs. If the bone marrow fails in its function, the patient dies. This need not be. The diseased or inadequate organ can be replaced, but doing so involves a long list of contingencies: A suitable bone marrow donor must be available. The patient must be able to withstand the preparatory treatment for a transplant. And then, if the graft takes, if the new marrow does not too severely attack the recipient's cells, if malignancies do not recur, and if infection does not win a race with the body's slowly returning immune system, the patient lives. A bone marrow transplant requires the dedication of a specialized physician[1] and of the patient and the patient's family, sophisticated technological facilities, and the resources of a large, well-staffed hospital.

Actually, the transplant begins before the patient and doctor meet. First, there's the assessment with the referring doctor. Rappeport worries about the phone calls he doesn't get—those about patients who could benefit from a transplant but whose doctors don't know about it or are prejudiced against it. He is highly critical of doctors who don't pursue the kind of therapy he offers; he dismisses as sentimental a doctor's concern about the social dislocation a child from a disturbed and disadvantaged family would experience receiving treatment far from home. The child might be saved, the child can be comforted, with the right care. The pediatrician in question might be worried—about the disease, about the patient— but not enough. "If he had enough angst, he'd call," says Rappeport. He is angry when, in his view, the child's doctor gives up prematurely. A bone marrow transplant should at least be considered—that is, talked over with someone prepared to implement it—in an instance when it is almost certainly the only chance at saving a young life.

"Now," says Rappeport, "anyone who needs a bone marrow transplant—in the United States—can get one." (This is wishful thinking on Rappeport's part. He's ignoring the fact that many people in the United States are without health insurance.) "But physicians don't know that. There used to be a struggle to get a patient treated; there were more candidates than there were beds. So you still often get calls that start, 'She's a very lovely person. The most lovely person you'll ever meet.' Sometimes there are fifty of the most lovely people you'll ever meet." Then the discussion gets down to actual indications: What disease does the patient have? What stage is it at? Does the patient have a donor? Is the patient receptive to the idea?

The understood value of a bone marrow transplant as therapy has changed and is broadening. Still, given the risks and sickness and the expense and the uncertain outcome of a specific transplant, what alternative therapies exist? And the hardest question for the patient to understand, Rappeport says, is: "Are the doctor and hospital he's approaching doing the particular kind of transplant he needs?" That is, do they have the experience and equipment for a given disease or variation on it? Is the institution one that has the right laboratory and personnel to treat the problems a specific marrow donation presents?

Next, Rappeport consults with other doctors, who vary according to a patient's condition—a pulmonary specialist for someone with lung disease, for example—who also understand bone marrow transplantation. Rappeport has to determine if a patient, sick though he may be, can withstand the rigors of a transplant. If someone dies as a result of the procedure, he says, whether or not the patient would have died anyway, it's his—Rappeport's—fault.

During their hospital stay, Rappeport's transplant patients receive their treatment—all but the irradiation—in laminar flow rooms, specially constructed sterile environments where the entire mass of filtered air is blown with uniform velocity along parallel flow lines. A yellow line on the room's floor marks the place beyond which only gowned, gloved, and masked visitors—including doctors and nurses—may step. Rubber gloves for examinations are built into a plastic curtain, equipped with a bubble through which visitors can speak, that separates the patient from the hall.[2]

Everything that goes into the room, from mail to communion wafers, is first sterilized. Everything is measured, everything noted. Medications, blood products, and—for the long periods of time the patient is too sick to eat—nutrients, too, are administered through central venous lines, which spare the patient the tortuous poking of multiple blood drawings and intravenous injections. (These lines, designed to allow easy access to the veins chemotherapy may have scarred, are devices, surgically implanted, tunneled through the skin directly to a vein that goes into the heart.)

The patient, each day, performs a sponge bath with twenty washcloths: He wipes down one side of his face, discards the cloth. Wipes the other side of his face, discards that cloth, and so on down his body. He smears antifungal ointments in his body's crevices. Four times a day, through what in Rappeport's practice is now, on the average, a six-week hospital stay, he swishes in his mouth, then swallows, a terrible-tasting nonabsorbable antibiotic—referred to as bowel prep—so that his gastrointestinal tract is sterile. Patients regularly cheat on this but never succeed in fooling the doctors and nurses for long: the bowel movements of people who take bowel prep don't have a foul odor.

At first, a nurse supervises the bath. Because of the necessity for constant, attentive patient care, Rappeport maintains, only partly disingenuously, that bone marrow transplantation is a nursing procedure. "I don't know how he'd feel about hearing this," says a nurse-clinician who has worked with Rappeport since the mid-seventies, "but Joel would make a great nurse. He's proud of how well they do," she says of Rappeport and his patients. "He doesn't care who he tells."

"You have to know where you stop and the patient begins," Rappeport says. One spring night, though, walking along a dark sidewalk, he keeps his voice even but turns his head away from me, because he is crying at the news he's learned and transmitted that afternoon: He's had to tell a young woman he'd tried to save that she's relapsed, and that means she is almost certainly in a hopeless situation now. He says each of "us"—the nurses and doctors—has to come to terms with death in his or her own way. He says his reaction to each person's death is different, that it's "like any circumstantial relationship you have in life." That once he kicked a hole in a door.

But leaning back from his desk, his hands clasped behind his head, Rappeport says, "What would you like to come out with in the end? You'd like to make a concrete contribution in some way, so that in the future some people will say, This is a contribution made by so-and-so, and it helps. And it helped X number of people. And I just think that's going to take, on my part, a lot of work."

The day-to-day reward comes in seeing patients well again, in the hematology outpatient clinic. "This is why I do it," he says. "To see them afterward. I don't know why, frankly, the nurses and house staff do it." He's speaking on a Tuesday, when post–bone marrow transplant patients return for the checkups that come twice weekly, weekly, biweekly, and eventually at yearly intervals. The clinic's a bustling place, full of frightened people. Many people wear blue paper surgical masks—the eyes above them always wary—and gloves, and pull back if a presumably germ-laden visitor comes too close.

Rappeport rushes from examining room to examining room. But with the patients, he becomes chatty and relaxed. He listens to hearts and lungs, he palpates abdomens. In a diagnostic procedure specific to his particular patients' history, he runs his hands along each one's skin, feeling for the lack of elasticity, the doughy consistency, that suggests graft-versus-host disease, a complication both peculiar to bone marrow transplantation and common to it. Rappeport's quick gesture—grasping a patient's arm, and stroking down it—looks affectionate and casual, but he's really concentrated and concerned. Graft-versus-host disease, along with the recurrence of the original illness and serious infection, are Rappeport's greatest posttransplant worries. He looks down throats and takes blood pressures. All the time, he talks and listens.

As with his lecture to medical students, Rappeport's clinic meetings with recovering and recovered patients, especially those he's known a long time, have a tone of cheerful intimacy. There's a sense of victory in having gotten this far and a reassurance in the ongoing nature of the conversations, all continuations of previous ones. Rappeport tells one patient how his blood counts compared with earlier ones, and another that there's a new study on the effect of gamma globulin. He's dictatorial, declaring that one young man can't go back to school until January. He's simultaneously absent-minded and focused with a woman in her midtwenties, interrupting his own superficial chat by telling her to "lie down while I feel your spleen." In one room he asks how the wedding plans are coming, and in another instructs a patient to eat only kosher cold cuts, "not the salami with the mold." Don't worry about the chicken pox the child of your mother's coworker came down with, Rappeport says to one patient, and still on the subject of infection, tells another that it's okay to swim in a private pool but not a public one, on the ocean side but not the bay side.

He covers the everyday: "How do you think the Red Sox are doing?" and, "Latex paint's fine to paint the house with, but not oil-based." Along with the sad and abnormal: "How's you father feeling?" he asks a transplant patient whose family has been doubly struck with cancer. And, "Once your liver's okay, we can give hormone replacement for the hot flashes," he says to an unmarried woman in her early thirties who is now, because of pretransplant irradiation, going through menopause.

There's problem after problem, but the word carries the implication of solution. Rappeport's happy. "We had five weddings last year," he says to me at the end of a clinic day. "We must be doing something right."

Rappeport first participated in a bone marrow transplant in 1964,[3] when he was a fourth-year medical student. Then, the patient immediately died. Now he cures half the people he treats with bone marrow transplants. The Rolodex on his desk is filled with the numbers and names of patients, which he writes in pencil because they move a lot. Bone marrow transplantation is still a therapy primarily for the young.

Many of these people still die—50 percent success means 50 percent failure. When I asked Rappeport how he stands all the people dying, he replied that a lot more people died when he started. And trying to explain further how he got into an area of medicine where death is everyday, and hope was once unlikely and is now tenuous, he lapses into a distant, almost editorial, delivery: "I guess my style is such that the decision had to do with trying to get people through this awful experience—curative chemotherapy, bone marrow transplants—we put them through."

Brian Smith says, "Joel's major motivation is a concern for the patients and a concern for trying to figure out what he can do on a technical level to alleviate the major clinical problems in hematology, but more specifically in bone marrow transplantation." Of Smith, Rappeport says, "I have fun with Brian. Not frivolous fun. Intellectual fun."

"Joel's object," says Smith, "is to be what we all give lip service to: the physician/scientist. To observe things at the bedside and then take them up to the laboratory and then back to the bedside again."

"I'm a doer," Rappeport says, "rather than a creator." How do you do a bone marrow transplant? "With meticulous attention to detail." What details? "Everything. Look, if you don't systematically look at—pick anything. How much urine the patient is producing. And you let that slide among the myriad of things that need to be done, you'll end up in trouble. Take anything. Magnesium levels." Seated at his desk, he leans forward, nods for emphasis. "If you pay attention assiduously to the urine output and happen to lapse on the magnesium level . . ." He sounds like Sondheim's Seurat: "Inch by inch . . ." Mandy Patinkin obsessively, passionately, placing the tiny dots of thousands of colors that, over the years, will become "Sunday on the Island of La Grand Jatte." "Bit by bit . . ."

An old mentor of Rappeport's says, "To do bone marrow transplants, you need persistence, and you need optimism."

On the morning of February 10, 1987, before classes, nineteen-year-old Wesley Fairfield went to the Bowdoin College Infirmary. He had had a cold and sore throat for a couple of weeks, and then a sore abdomen. Then he started to run a fever and had sores in his mouth. Dr. Roy Weymouth, who coincidentally had been a medical school classmate of Rappeport's, knew right away that Wesley had leukemia. Identification of the subgroup—and the disease has many—came later, after laboratory tests. But even at the initial examination Weymouth could tell that Wesley was seriously ill. Most threatening, to Weymouth's eye, was Wesley's extreme pallor. "I asked Wesley if he had anything else to show me, any bruises, and he showed me discolorations on his shins. I was sure." He drew blood, put Wes to bed, and waited for the pathologist's call.

The word *leukemia* describes a large group of diseases that afflict a relatively small number of people—in the United States about 20,000 people a year are diagnosed with it. Leukemias and lymphomas are among the "liquid tumors" in which hematologists specialize. Unlike oncologists, however, hematologists do not restrict themselves to malignant disease. They also treat people with anemia, a word that describes insufficiencies and disorders of the red cell, and clotting problems such as hemophilia. Often, individual hematologists concentrate on one or another category within the broad spectrum of blood diseases.

In addition to cancer and anemia and bleeding disorders, there is a wide range of illnesses where one or another blood component, instead of failing in its function, overdoes it, seeping and exploding into the function or turf of other body parts, so that the skin turns orange or green, erupts or festers, bones break, infections proliferate, growth is stunted. Some of these diseases are hereditary, and even in those that are not, there's often an identifiable genetic component—chromosomal change detectable under a microscope—that is sometimes, as in most of the leukemias, incompletely understood. In many of the most interesting and devastating diseases hematologists address, immune function is severely compromised or nonexistent. Sometimes the diseases overlap: What seems to be sickle cell anemia could be thalassemia; aplastic anemia can turn into leukemia.

An hour after Roy Weymouth finished examining Wesley, confirmation came from the pathologists, and Weymouth first told Wesley and then the family. Martha Fairfield, Wesley's mother, was at work, in her glass-walled office at a bank. "Dr. Weymouth said, 'It's either aplastic anemia or leukemia.' I started to cry, and my office is a fishbowl—I hung up and called him back from somewhere else."

"I hated having to tell the Fairfields that way," Weymouth says. "Over the phone. What do you say? How do you start the conversation? I tossed it over and over and over in my mind." Weymouth had Wesley's twin brother Scott, also a Bowdoin student, pulled out of class.

"I asked Dr. Weymouth if Wes was going to die," Scott said, "and he said he didn't know." The brothers—muscular and sweet-faced, with thick, longish black hair and, in Wesley's case, glasses—didn't say anything. "They just folded into each other's arms," Weymouth said. "They were like one. Scott was more visibly shaken than his brother. Wes was trying to keep Scott together. We all cried." Early the following September, on a sunny warm morning, Weymouth cried again, remembering it.

The Bowdoin infirmary is shadowy but safe: big, square nineteenth-century rooms, mottled green linoleum on the floor, high white beds. It's a place students go with a broken arm or a case of the grippe.

"Wesley's a tough kid," Weymouth said. "It's a strange term for somebody who's so gentle. But he wanted to go to class. He didn't want to be put to bed. A good old Yankee, I'll tell you. We don't see many students like that."

Wesley's leukemia was the first case Weymouth had seen in twelve years of college medicine. As soon as Weymouth had the diagnosis, he arranged for Wesley to be admitted to Massachusetts General Hospital, in Boston, where he could receive the care he needed. Wesley and Scott, driving the old car that they shared, left right away. "I remember I sat down and drew them a map," Weymouth said. "I hated to send them off that way, alone. But there was no time to be lost."

"Dr. Weymouth wanted us on the road by one," Scott said. "We didn't talk much on the ride down to Boston." Weymouth's judgment was excellent. Wesley had acute (*acute* in medical terminology meaning not only "intense," as it does in ordinary usage, but also "of fast onset") myelogenous leukemia. A delay in treatment could have been fatal.

By five that winter afternoon, Wesley had been admitted to the Mass General. Martha and Ed Fairfield, driving from western Massachusetts, arrived shortly after their sons and, in the huge parking garage, happened to pull in right next to their sons' car. They rushed to the emergency room. There, as soon as the doctors saw Scott—identical in looks to Wesley—they started talking transplant. But first, to get the remission that would make a successful transplant more probable, there were weeks of chemotherapy. Wesley ran a high fever, evidence of an infection, one that wouldn't respond to medication.

And then, a week into treatment, massive bleeding from Wesley's bowel, and surgery. "They hoped they could stop the bleeding," Martha Fairfield said. "But they weren't sure exactly where it was coming from. They said he might need a colostomy, maybe permanently." The doctors said their operating table was the safest place for Wesley to be.

"But they don't say why you're there," Wesley said. Surgeons found the cause of the bleeding and stopped it. There was no colostomy. Over forty Dekes—Scott and Wesley's fraternity, some of them young women, all called brothers—traveled down to Boston to give blood.

In leukemia, abnormal blood cells multiply, eventually crowding out those that behave normally. Bone marrow usually generates orderly, geometric blood growth, starting with the stem cell and progressing through intermediate cells to differentiated cells, each dedicated to a preordained and critical task. When a person suffers from leukemia, his or her bone marrow produces a disproportionate quantity of weak, malformed, ineffectual, and yet overwhelming white blood cells. The leukemic cells don't grow as well as normal ones, but they *don't stop*. These two facts explain both why leukemia commonly kills and why chemotherapy can sometimes defeat it.

"Normal cells stop proliferating when there are enough cells around," says Brian Smith, "but leukemic cells will never stop, so that even if they're not quite as good as the normal cells, they eventually win. Because they just never quit." The problem, says Smith, is that all the chemotherapeutic drugs commonly used for leukemia kill off the normal cells along with the abnormal ones. "They apparently do a slightly better job on the leukemic cells, because fortunately, in some leukemias—childhood ALL [acute lymphatic leukemia] for instance—80 percent or so of kids can be cured. But still, the issue remains that leukemic cells kill because they don't know when to quit, and not because they are intrinsically much tougher or much more resilient cells than normal cells.

"If you could find something unique to the leukemic cell and target that," leaving the normal cells alone, "you could presumably kill off the leukemic one better—because you'd be more specific at it—and also with a lot fewer side effects." In this widely desired and worked-toward scenario, "the horrible side effects of chemotherapy—the obvious ones, like feeling sick to your stomach and throwing up and hair falling out, and the less apparent side effects that can be fatal: blood counts (platelets and white cells and so on) going down—would not occur. Those things are really due to the fact that we can't target the cell we want to target specifically. When we try to kill the leukemic cell, all we have is a drug that kills cells that are dividing real fast. And cells that are dividing real fast include hair cells, cells in your gastrointestinal tract, and the normal bone marrow cells. So what happens? The hair falls out, the stomach cells fall out and make you vomit, the bone marrow cells fall out temporarily and make your blood counts go down."

"Wes and I don't remember that time very well," Scott says, speaking of Wesley's initial bout with chemotherapy. The Mass General hospitalization lasted for four weeks. Martha talked to Roy Weymouth every day. For transplantation, she said, "Dr. Rappeport's name was the first, the last, the only one mentioned. Dr. Weymouth said he was world-famous."

The two doctors hadn't been close friends in medical school, but Weymouth remembered Rappeport from that time. Ten years after they'd graduated, Weymouth turned on "Agronsky and Company" and "There was Joel talking about bone marrow transplants. I was astounded. I knew what he was doing, but I hadn't realized his prominence. Joel was an excellent student, but not a bore, not a grind. He had a good sense of humor. I don't think there was anyone in the class who didn't enjoy being around him and respect him as well. At that point, everybody's pretty much the same. You have no idea who's going to migrate to the top of their fields. Joel was a very good medical student, but there was nothing that indicated he'd be leading a major program of this nature."

The Fairfields first met Rappeport March 27, 1987. They all liked him right away. Ed Fairfield says, "Dr. Rappeport's disheveledness makes him look caring about his work, and his work is the patient. I like the fact he's disheveled. Because I'm disheveled too, I guess." Nevertheless, this initial meeting was, as these always are, terrifying.

Wesley, now in remission, had thought the worst was behind him. "They don't tell you that you're over the hill but the mountain's still ahead," he says. He heard about the mountain that day, as he sat, with his parents and Scott, the prospective donor, in Rappeport's office. The room has a computer and shelves of medical books, many of them loose-leaf notebooks with current information on transplantation centers, drugs, and biological modifiers. Rappeport had hung up maps, aerial views of his beloved Lake Winnipesaukee, and autographed photos of his mentors. There is a plaster model of an airplane a young patient had painted—yellow and blue, red and green—with the insignia LAF (for laminar air flow, the special system that cleans the air of bone marrow transplant hospital rooms). The office is a bright corner room, but it's a grim place for anyone who must listen to what Rappeport has to say during an informed-consent meeting.

In his discussion with the Fairfields, Rappeport did what he always does in these conversations. He not only explained to the family what was to happen, he also made sure they understood the danger. When a bone marrow transplant is used for malignant disease, it is basically a rescue mission. Because healthy marrow—the donor's—is available to the patient, it is possible to use huge doses of chemotherapeutic drugs and radiation that completely destroy the recipient's marrow. If it were not for the new marrow that is to come, the patient would definitely die from the preparatory treatment. "They kill you, then they bring you back to life," my sister Roberta said.

"Hearing what could go wrong in a transplant—that was scary," Wesley said. "Then Dr. Rappeport said he wanted to ask *me* a question. He asked me if I understood what would happen if the transplant didn't work. I didn't get him at first. And I said, 'Then there'll be more chemotherapy.' And he said, 'Well, let's assume that doesn't work.' I didn't know what he was looking for, and I finally realized he was asking if I understood that it's fatal. That was hard."

The difficulty of bone marrow transplantation today lies in the preparation of the patient and of the marrow and, most of all, in the judgment and watchfulness required ahead of time, through the weeks of hospitalization, through the year or more of near-isolation at home, and in the lifelong necessity for specialized medical monitoring.

The science that supports bone marrow transplantation goes back to the fifties, when the first transplants—on mice, still the magical scientific animal—were performed, an outgrowth of research on atomic energy, as part of the Manhattan Project. Today, knowledge and technology are mushrooming, not only with the broadening of donor-recipient matches but also with the help of new substances that make possible the growth of small numbers of stem cells in test tubes. Through the use of blood taken from fetal umbilical cords, it may be possible to obtain enough cells for a transplant, especially when they are amplified with the new biological modifiers that increase cell production. Nevertheless, except for autologous transplants—those in which the patient's own marrow is used after an effort to eradicate diseased cells—all transplants require a donor.

"A very interesting thing to think about," says Rappeport, "is that pregnancy is really temporary transplantation. It can be thought of as the ultimate rejection. Not psychologically—immunologically. And why there aren't more chronic aborters doesn't make sense. You would think that after five or six kids, for example, a woman would have an immune response against the fetus. In some chronic aborters that happens to be the problem: they have antibodies, an immune defense, against their husbands' genetic material. God didn't give us transplantation antigens so we would be able to reject someone's kidney. HLA material [antigens of the histo-compatible locus, the genetic area—on chromosome 6—where donor and recipient must match] is probably part of the normal immune response. There must be a reason in terms of conservation of the species, which isn't obvious right now."

Because Wesley is an identical twin, it was a virtual certainty that his body would not reject Scott's marrow, and almost impossible that the new marrow would attack his own organs. The latter phenomenon, called graft-versus-host disease, is a terrible, sometimes lethal, complication of bone marrow transplants that can occur when there is an imperfect genetic match between recipient and donor. For Wesley, knowledge that he wouldn't get graft-versus-host disease (GVH) was not an unmitigated comfort: Some GVH works against leukemic relapse. The removal of one risk increases another. The decision to have the transplant, however, Martha Fairfield says, was Wesley's.

"The numbers," said Scott, referring to the 50 to 60 percent chance of cure Wes had with a bone marrow transplant versus a 20 percent chance with chemotherapy alone, "were staggering." (Wesley is the only patient I describe in this book for whom treatment other than a bone marrow transplant held out *any* hope of cure.)

Wesley was forceful in his response: "I wanted it."

The bone marrow transplant consent form, the contents of which Rappeport explains and expands on, always at length and repeatedly, is a terrifying document. In four single-spaced computer-printed pages it describes, often in technical terms, the radiation and chemotherapeutic preparation and the transplantation procedure itself, including any experimental aspects. It then lists the dangers, in two long paragraphs starting with the sentence, "The risks of the procedure to you are extreme." If the graft doesn't take, the preparatory drugs and irradiation are lethal, since the patient's own bone marrow will by then have been destroyed. Even if the graft does take, there will be hair loss and vomiting. There may be dry mouth, fever, jaw pain, and lung damage. Irradiation will cause sterility and may cause cataracts. There may be bladder bleeding, mouth ulcers (which can be so painful that the patient needs morphine in order to swallow his own saliva), skin rashes, liver disease, and eye inflammation. Even before the transplant, there could be a fatal reaction to a preparatory drug.

After the transplant, the consent form goes on, dangers continue. Engraftment may appear to have occurred and then fail, resulting in certain death. The graft may react against the patient, causing graft-versus-host disease, which, the form states, chiefly affects the skin, the liver, and the gut and which can be mild or severe, chronic or acute, and which can kill.

The destruction of patients' immune systems leaves them vulnerable for months. For at least a year, Rappeport's patients are on low-bacteria diets (no peanuts, fresh vegetables, fruit, or shellfish); although they stop taking bowel prep when they leave the hospital their own gastrointestinal bacteria are still a threat. Patients have to maintain scrupulous personal hygiene and are not allowed sex. The last is a rule patients confess to breaking, and then feeling terrible guilt at the risk they've incurred. Once home, until immune function returns, patients—even in surgical masks and gloves—are allowed few visitors and virtually no visits. "House arrest," the husband of one patient calls it. All necessary because an infection—even a cold—could kill, in the absence of a normal immune system.[4] For Wesley, this meant he wouldn't be able to go back to Bowdoin for a year. Pneumocystis and CMV (cytomegalovirus) pneumonia—the same infections that afflict AIDS patients—are a strong possibility in the immediate posttransplant months. (Bone marrow transplants cannot cure AIDS because there is no way, at this time, to eradicate the virus that causes the disease.) If there is pneumonia, there may be permanent lung damage or death.

During hospitalization, there will be more bone marrow aspirations, and pain. There will be from ten to a hundred transfusions of red blood cells and other blood components, especially platelets. Transfusion (despite specially irradiated blood products, processed in a way used only for bone marrow transplant patients, patients on immunosuppressive drugs, fetuses, and tiny newborns) creates a risk of hepatitis, of cytomegalovirus (again, dangerous specifically to people with suppressed immune systems), and of other infections. In the hospital and afterward, herpes zoster (shingles) is nearly universal in people who have previously had chicken pox, and herpes simplex (the cold sore virus) is common but—since the development in the late 1970s of the antiviral drug acyclovir—not fatal.

The heart may be damaged. There may also be low blood pressure, joint pain, liver and kidney damage. There is an increased risk of tumors later in life. Leukemia could recur. The consent form says, too, that the long-term effects of some of the drugs are largely unknown. All this the Fairfields heard and read, and Rappeport explained, before the transplant.

At this first meeting Rappeport told Wesley that chemotherapy and radiation were an effort to wipe out leukemic cells, but that there was a level below which accurate measurement wasn't possible. That is, though the treatment is intended to destroy the marrow completely, some undetectable cells, including leukemic ones, may remain.

"I asked him," Wesley said, " 'How much do you know about these measurements?' and he said, 'It's crude.' And that scared me."

"It was *terrible*," says Scott, referring to the whole meeting. A little later, though, he reconsiders his judgment. "It was good. Because it showed us not only what Dr. Rappeport knew but also that he'd be straight with us, he'd be square with us. And he was."

"That's the point," Rappeport says. "To establish trust."

Nevertheless, Wesley says, "You can't picture it, unless you've been through it, because you can't picture the fear." But, he says, "The hope subdues the fear."

After that first meeting, out in the hall, "Dr. Rappeport beckoned me over," Wesley said. "He looked very serious. 'Come over here,' he said. 'Bring your brother.' I thought he had something very serious to tell us. He took us over to a little room and pointed to a plate of chocolate chip cookies and ate one and told us to have one. He likes sweets. At least, I think he does."

Scott Fairfield, a biology major, talks with fluency about milligrams of doses, logs of measurements. But Wesley says before he got leukemia, all either he or his brother knew about it was the word. And Scott says he didn't know how to spell that. When asked about being a donor, his voice fades. He admits his hips were sore afterward, but "compared to what Wes was going through . . ."

A bone marrow transplant is not an "operation" in the usual sense. There is no surgery. It is unlike solid organ transplants—those of the heart, liver, kidney, and pancreas—in that way. It is

also different in that the donor is always living and is left un-
harmed, because bone marrow regenerates. Most strikingly, a bone
marrow transplant is different from others in that when the procedure is fully successful, the organ functions completely as one's
own. Once that's happened, the patient no longer requires immunosuppressive drugs in order to tolerate the acquired marrow.

After chemotherapy and—sometimes—radiation destroy the
patient's own bone marrow, the donor's is taken from the pelvis
through hundreds of aspirations; that is, the removal by suction
through needles and syringes. This is the only part of a bone marrow transplant that looks the way doctor dramas, both actual and
fictional, have taught us to imagine cutting-edge medicine. It is
called a "harvest," an accurate but incongruous term; the almost
certainly scared and worried donor isn't a wheat field. For Rappeport, a marrow harvest is a frequent event but also a highly
unusual one, in that while it is taking place, the emotional side of
patient care is nonexistent. Hematologists are internists, not surgeons, and their work as clinicians involves thinking and talking,
not cutting or on-the-spot reordering of anyone's anatomy. Indeed,
the person on the table, though in Rappeport's care for a few hours,
isn't his primary patient. The person whose illness has brought him
to Rappeport is in another part of the hospital, in a laminar flow
room, awaiting the marrow infusion.

For a typical harvest, Rappeport and Smith scrub at a sink
outside the operating room. There is, as is usual in proceedings
involving Rappeport, an entourage—in this case, junior doctors[5]
and nurses new to the bone marrow transplant unit. All of them
cover their arms first with bright yellow suds, then—from a different kind of soap—pink. Around the corner from the sink, a
three-year-old donor is made unconscious. A few minutes earlier,
in the holding area outside the operating rooms, she'd been crying,
probably from hunger; she wasn't allowed to eat before receiving
anesthesia, and the marrow harvest, scheduled for one o'clock, is
taking place at four, because a kidney transplant took longer than
anticipated, disrupting the operating room schedule.

The donor's parents have spent the whole day trying to calm
and distract their little girl. It is a terrible time for them, the worst
they've had to go through, because they have two children in the
hospital at once. In addition to the three-year-old, there's the recipient. He's a seven-year-old boy, now lying, devoid of immunity,
in bed in his sterile hospital room.

In the operating room, before the doctors and nurses take turns aspirating marrow, Brian Smith checks the metal canisters into which it will be placed. Each contains an anticoagulant, and they are lined up with much of the rest of the equipment for the harvest on a high, narrow, blue-draped table at one end of the room. The table, with its carefully arranged syringes and needles, its sterile receptacles, its special fluid solutions, the plastic bag with a long tube from which the marrow will be infused into the patient, and the test tubes that will hold additional marrow for laboratory use, looks like an altar, prepared for Mass. Smith, a Catholic, says it looks like a table to him. Rappeport, who checked everyone's glove sizes outside, says he'll prep, and swabs the donor with antiseptic. The nurse in charge of the operating room tells a resident to take off his wedding ring and scrub for three more minutes. The anesthesiologist, hoarse from a long day at the crucial head of the table, suctions the little girl's throat, tapes her eyelids shut, and watches the colored, beeping monitors. A tube in the child's esophagus goes to the anesthesiologist's ear, making it possible for the doctor to hear the donor's breathing and heart sounds.

Rappeport, Smith, and their trainees attach needles to syringes, plunge them into the donor's posterior iliac crest—the pelvic bone in her rear end, the only undraped part of her body except her head, now in the care of the anesthesiologist and her assistants—and yank them out again. It takes strength to pull the marrow, even from a toddler's body, and the nurses and doctors work in relays. A nurse's hands tremble slightly; she's done this before, but never on a child.

Though the risk to the donor is negligible, almost nonexistent —and, as Scott says, in the face of the possible good of the recipient, irrelevant—there is discomfort, some of it perhaps avoidable. Years after I served as a donor, I have twinges of pain in the pelvic area from which marrow was drawn; I wonder how experienced or careful someone who aspirated it from me was. Furthermore, and less dismissible, I was exhausted from the time of my donation until the marrow regenerated—a matter of weeks, during a period of great emotional distress. I had asked Rappeport, well ahead of time, if I should donate my own blood in advance, so I could receive it as a transfusion at the time of the transplant. He told me it wasn't necessary, and continues to refuse to employ the practice, saying no donor has ever needed a transfusion. Need, in this instance, is a matter of interpretation. Though it's no doubt true that none of

Rappeport's patients' donors have required medical care because of marrow depletion, it is also the case that autologous blood transfusion would, with virtually no risk, make them—us—feel better quicker.

The marrow usually comes out the color of strawberry Jell-O, but some aspirations are darker than others. Rappeport has no explanation for this. The foam is fat. Every time someone fills a syringe, he or she hands it to a colleague, who empties it into one of the canisters, first removing the needle so as to avoid breaking up cells, then attaching a new one and handing the syringe back. The needles are long and thick—they look like awls—but they're inserted in the same places in the skin over and over again. The donor will be left with few, tiny, and nearly invisible scars. Everything about the routine is smooth, efficient, and calm. Throughout, a nurse writes notes into a chart. At the end the anesthesiologist pulls the tube from the donor's throat, suctions her again, takes the tape off her eyes, swabs her bottom with antiseptic, and injects a sedative.

All through the procedure, and starting outside at the sinks, there's casual conversation, some of it jokes, some of it business. Smith and Rappeport, in particular, talk about treating the marrow. If there's little genetic disparity, as with these children, or presumably none, as with Wesley and Scott, and if the recipient is young, the marrow is simply strained, to remove clumps and bone chips.

But if the patient is older,[6] and sometimes, if the donor and recipient are of different sexes, or if there is significant genetic dissimilarity between them at the critical HLA locus,[7] the marrow might be treated to reduce the probable severity of graft-versus-host disease. Smith has just heard that Memorial Sloan-Kettering Cancer Center, in New York, is treating the marrow of unrelated donors, and he and Rappeport chat about the methodologies and trade-offs of various techniques. Making marrow from more donors efficacious for more recipients is critical to the extension and success of bone marrow transplantation. In a few months Smith will go to New York to learn the techniques used there and, with Rappeport, weigh them against those they've used in the past and those now in the offing.

Regardless of what is or isn't done to the marrow, it's given as a blood transfusion. It will be days or weeks before the marrow migrates to the bones' cavities, where it will begin, from the essen-

tial pluripotent stem cell (or progenitor cell), to produce red cells
and white cells in all their variety, and platelets, so there is nothing
dramatic to see. Still, most patients are emotional about the infusion. And although a bone marrow transplant really takes place
over months, neither donor nor recipient forgets the date of the
infusion. Rappeport himself is relieved when the donor's marrow is
actually in his patient's body.

During his hospitalization Wesley, afraid of contamination,
didn't want any visitors in his room. He preferred to see them
outside the plastic curtain (where they would be in their street
clothes, rather than gowned and masked) and to talk to them
through the bubble. Scott spent all day, every day, with his
brother. "Just to have family there," Wesley said. "Even if you're
sleeping, knowing they're there helps."

Wesley was terribly embarrassed at the nurse's initial supervision of his sponge bath. But at the same time, "Losing my sense
of privacy almost made me closer to the nurses. Having no sense of
privacy, I felt I could talk about anything. And did. We would sit
there, and when they were in the room for an hour and a half or so,
I'd talk about anything and really get to know them. Especially in
those flow rooms, because they come up to the screen and talk to
you all the time. The nurses are friendly with you, but they're
always doing their job. If you say you think your throat hurts
maybe a little, she may not seem to be paying attention, but she's
always very, very careful—the next thing you know there's a doctor
looking down your throat."

"The people you work with," says Carol McGarigle, a nurse
who worked with Rappeport for fifteen years, "are the only people
who can understand what you're going through—about what you're
doing and about supporting the patients, and about what the patients feel. No one else ever gets to know exactly what it feels like,
and it is hard to describe. You work closely with somebody for a
long period of time, and you have this sense of they'll take care of
this, and I'll take care of that, and it gets done, but you don't talk
about it. That kind of relationship creates the atmosphere that
keeps people doing their jobs very well. You want nurses who
really want to be here, who are committed to this kind of patient
care, and are willing to spend the time and emotional investment in
doing it. It can't be a job; it can't be an eight-hour-a-day job if it's
going to work well."

Brian Smith says, "Most bone marrow transplant units have

an extremely short half-life for nurses." He's borrowed the scientific term that describes the length of a substance's efficacy. "Six months and they quit." The strain is too great for most people.

Wesley is grateful that because Scott's genetically identical marrow wouldn't attack his cells, he was spared the horror of graft-versus-host disease. He had fevers and fear and vomiting. But compared with what other people were going through, he felt lucky.

"I guess the thing that made it not so bad for me was that I was basically coasting through—with the exception of my high fevers—with no complications. No graft-versus-host. And the guy two rooms down, his liver was not functioning, and everybody else was having graft-versus-host. I was in the center room—and you know, you keep track of how the other patients are doing, and they're always struggling. One guy was there 105 days and got out a few weeks *after* I left. There was Thomas, who didn't make it. And somebody else died quickly. Relative to their experience I felt like I was just coasting through the transplant."

By summer, he was home. There, he worked with his computer, read, and exercised. Scott went back to school in the fall, and Martha and Ed returned full-time to their jobs; both their employers had been understanding and supportive during all the time of Wesley's illness. Wesley showed not only fortitude but maturity. He kept himself occupied but was careful to preserve himself—conscientiously smearing himself with the sunscreen his radiation-exposed skin needs when he goes outside and wearing a surgical mask when, in January, he enrolled in a couple of classes at the college in his town. When I visited the Fairfields, there wasn't a speck of dust, and their house—scrubbed daily, according to the rules—smelled like a swimming pool.

It worked; everything went as it should. Although Wesley became dehydrated shortly after he was released from the hospital, and had to return for a few days, he suffered no complications. The following September he returned to Bowdoin, graduating only a semester after his brother.

On a rainy November day during their senior year Scott, almost finished at college, says good things did come out of Wesley's experience and his. He is diffident, expressing his feelings. "I figured out what's important to me, I guess. Things like the blood drive," the one that he's organized, the statistics of which he quotes with pride. "Like helping people," his voice dropping as he says that. "How important the family is. And friends." He twists his napkin to shreds, though, eating lunch in his fraternity house.

"I'm always looking at Wes's skin color, looking for that paleness that was there before. When it happened, I didn't suspect what it was, but I remember looking at him and thinking, God, he's pale. Now, I'm always telling him when he looks tired. When I look at him now and he's tired, I don't think, Oh, he's tired. I think, How's he feeling? It's like I'm watching over him. It's hard to know if our relationship has changed because of the transplant, because over time your relationship changes anyway. But I'm definitely more protective. For instance, he's very involved with his girlfriend, and I'm always telling him to be careful, because I'd hate to see him have his feelings get hurt."

In a basement laboratory a few buildings away from the fraternity house, Wesley, surrounded by scientific equipment, works on the experiment that's part of the honors program he's completing. He says he's the happiest he's ever been, that he's doing well academically and has a wonderful girlfriend. He can't say he's closer to Scott than he was before, because they were so close to start with, but they bicker less. He says he no longer thinks of his illness and the transplant every day, but there are reminders: His experiment is on lobsters, and he can't eat shellfish. He always wears slippers and tries never to have his bare feet touch the floor. He washes his hands a lot. People failing to cover their mouths and noses when they cough and sneeze, Wes says, "really gets me." But of the whole experience, he says, "I think a lot of good has come of it. I don't look back and say it's a terrible experience; I say it's a growing experience. I think it's changed me in a lot of ways, but I don't feel I've changed. I've changed the way I look at things—my eyes are more open to my life. It's hard to explain," says Wes. "But I don't get as sad for as long. Everything's in a different perspective—the horrible things aren't as horrible anymore. Horrible isn't the right word," he says. "It's that the same circumstances that would have irritated or depressed me don't now—or not for long." He says he'd like to be a doctor, probably a hematologist, probably do bone marrow transplants—because who could understand the patient's dilemmas better than he?

Why, in the sixties, did Rappeport decide on hematology? Why on bone marrow transplantation, before it was a successful therapy? "During the second year of my residency I didn't know exactly what I wanted to do. I wanted to take care of sick patients and make some clinical impact. I didn't consciously blend high-tech and general practice, because at that time there was basically no high-tech. But my father—a GP—told me very clearly that there was a hierarchy in medicine."

Rappeport's father Arthur was a twenty-four-hour-a-day, seven-days-a-week doctor. "Grouchy but nice," as a worker in the elder Rappeport's Quincy, Massachusetts, hospital remembers him. "Joel's a lot like his father," says Linda, the younger Rappeport's wife. "He doesn't like to hear it, though."

Rappeport doesn't emphasize the impact of his early experience, but its obvious influence has to have been enormous. He remembers his father taking him on house calls, and patients—or their wives or mothers—inviting him in for a piece of pie. The patients always came first. His father's office was in the Rappeports' house; Joel remembers patients arriving for evening office hours earlier and earlier, and the family dinner being moved accordingly. Joel's sister Muriel remembers the family being packed and dressed and on their way out the door for a vacation, but turning around when a patient called. A friend of Joel's remembers that at Arthur Rappeport's funeral, the rabbi's only comment about Joel and Muriel was that "one became a doctor, and the other married a doctor." Rappeport says now that he considered other occupations, but his childhood friends and grade school and high school teachers assumed he would be a doctor. Many people can't imagine him being anything else.

The Rappeport family was proud and respected. Rose Rappeport, Joel's mother, was known for her good works and her beauty—her hats were famous—and was and is intent on maintaining her family's unalloyed positive public image. One of the tenets Rappeport most often quotes from his childhood is his mother's injunction "not to wash your dirty linen in public." The other was his father's insistence on the division between groups of people: "It was always us and them, us and them." Rappeport claims that when he was growing up, he heard this every day. Arthur Rappeport was talking about Jews and Gentiles. Joel doesn't seem alienated from non-Jews, but he's retained the principle. "We," he says today, categorizing doctors, or the staff and patients on the bone marrow transplant unit, or hematologists, in the course of pointing out, or just assuming, a difference—usually a moral superiority, always a defensive position—between the groups with which he's identifying himself and everyone else. He doesn't hear the implicit "they." Private doctors are different from, and largely in opposition to, academicians such as himself. So are hospital administrators.

Rappeport learned pride and defensiveness from his parents, but they also gave him a strong ethical sense and a feeling of obligation to help other people.

In elementary school and high school, Rappeport was completely successful. He was an excellent student whom teachers remember for his pure intellectual curiosity. His fourth-grade teacher told me Joel would cross a playing field to ask a question, and Bob Burdett, Rappeport's high school science teacher, says that Joel was a teacher's dream, the student who doesn't care about grades but just wants to learn. He was also a football player and president of the student council.

After high school, Rappeport went to Yale and then to Tufts Medical School in Boston. He got married—to a young woman he'd known all his life—after his first year in medical school, and within a few years had two children, a boy and a girl. His family life remains stable, but he spends very little time with his wife and children. He settled the facts of his life early and hasn't deviated from the traditional personal course he chose.

Rappeport's son Steven told me his father seems more comfortable at the hospital than anywhere else. Rappeport took umbrage at this view, but I agree with it. At the hospital, he has the constant—to someone else, the unremitting—opportunity to take or discuss an action related to his profession. "He's great for what you call a schmooz," a New Zealand hematologist, living in Boston, told me. Whether the topic is a patient or the trials of dealing with bureaucracy, or his or someone else's job dissatisfaction, escape from boredom and isolation is always possible in his workplace, one that functions twenty-four hours every day.

It is not true, as patients assume, that it is his effort to solve pressing medical problems that always gives Rappeport his distracted air. The repetitive minutiae present in all working lives constantly gnaw at him. He responds to inconvenience as if it were injustice, reacting with startling rudeness: He frequently initiates telephone calls while someone is in his office talking to him, he interrupts conversations with streams of complaints that have no relevance to the topic at hand, and he assumes his time is more valuable than that of other people.

Though Rappeport retains his idealism, he also has a kind of simpleminded competitiveness. To indicate the intelligence of colleagues, for example, he's bragged to me about their College Board scores, and seems unconscious of the inappropriateness of a group of grown men and women competing about these numbers decades after the fact. Rappeport assumes respect is due people who meet the most narrow, traditional, and widely acknowledged standard: male doctors who occupy positions of power in the institutions and specialties he's accustomed to revering. He doesn't know where the phrase "genealogy of training" originated, but he loves it, wanting to be part of a historic flow of earned trust.

"In medical school," Rappeport says, "it was pointed out that academic medicine was far superior to the practice of primary care. And then, I'd been an English lit major, I knew how to read a book, knew how to write a critical paper, and that was about it, so during my summer vacation, first year in medical school, I decided that I'd better try to work in a laboratory and find out what this was all about." He got a job in the lab of Robert Schwartz, now head of hematology at Tufts–New England Medical Center, who then worked for Dr. William Dameshek. "And Dameshek had this very vibrant department. It was large, but it was very exciting. And I think there are a number of things, not all of which are rational, which end up making your choice. Some teacher influenced you. And in this particular instance it was Bob Schwartz and Dr. Dameshek. And then, three years later, when I was a fourth-year student, I had a clinical hematology rotation, and I was sent to work up a patient one day, and it turned out to be my favorite teacher from high school, who had developed aplastic anemia from a relatively new drug. I was involved in his care, and subsequently whenever he was in the hospital I'd come visit him, and when he died I was sort of devastated. Aplastic anemia was one of the first diseases treated by bone marrow transplantation.

"During the second year of my residency I didn't know exactly what I wanted to do. Knew it was hematology, knew I wanted to take care of patients within that sphere. I had no illusions about wanting to do benchwork [laboratory science], however. I wanted to go where they had the best clinical program and took care of sick patients, at a time when malignancy was still a dirty word. But steps were evolving, and there was the issue: they needed someone to take care of them. You can't shoot 'em. You could, but you can't," he amends scrupulously. "It was not infrequent, in that particular time, to have the general practitioner or internist or surgeon call up and literally cry on the phone, 'Will you please tell my patient because I don't want to.' There was this whole void. Plus, you knew—things were going to change. No one had any idea what the rate would be. It certainly has not been fast, but there have been definite areas of progress."

The critical fact about Rappeport is the choice he made—and has stuck to—to try to save lives other people give up on. When he went to work at the Peter Bent Brigham Hospital (now the Brigham and Women's Hospital), there was no bone marrow transplant program in Boston. (Now, major university-affiliated medical centers often require them, for teaching and research purposes as much as for therapeutic ones.) Rappeport was assigned work he didn't much like, and one day walked from the Brigham to Children's Hospital next door, where there sat, still crated, a white cell harvester. It had been there, in its box, for months, "because there was no one interested in uncrating it and looking at the instructions, and certainly not in running it, so I went over and did it. Because a lot of our patients were dying of infections, and this was a clinical tool one could use, where you could start having perhaps some impact on patient survival."

The white blood cells called granulocytes help fight infection, and it is infections or hemorrhaging or both that kill people with leukemia. When Rappeport began, white blood cells from people with chronic leukemia were given to people with the acute forms of the disease since, for the latter, anything was an improvement over their existing condition. Today, this is not done. Now that there is curative therapy for people with leukemia, it is inappropriate to replace one disease with another, and in any case, there is a limit to the white blood cells a person, even one with the overabundance of chronic leukemia, can supply. Also, the blessings of more, and more sophisticated, antibiotics make granulocyte transfusions from any source largely passé.

"And so," Rappeport says, harking back to his cell separator experience, "when a transplant program was proposed, and the board of trustees agreed to it, and they needed white cell support for a transplant program, I was invited to help."

Dr. William Moloney tried to discourage him. "I didn't think it would work," he says today.

But it was Moloney whose presence had drawn Rappeport to the Brigham in the first place. Moloney had been caring for people with leukemia from the start of his own career, in the era before antibiotics. His first scientific paper dealt with leukemics dying of infections following tooth extractions. These deaths, he points out with force—Moloney, in his eighties and after a lifetime of looking at sickness and dying, is still emotionally involved in everything he talks about—came as a shock to the dentists who unwittingly provoked them. They weren't used to their patients dying. He was, though. When a patient was dying, Moloney went to the sick person's house and stayed there until he or she did die. He remembers that the untreatable infections sometimes smelled so bad it was hard to walk into the sickroom. Moloney was an ideal doctor. He is proud of having done everything possible for his patients, but he is completely unsentimental about the limitations of what he was able to do.

For a long, long time he could not offer them even the hope of recovery. The family and doctor were there—Moloney knows he did what was right—but death was inevitable and sickness dreadful and disgusting. Moloney's memories provide a fine jolt of realism, an antidote to notions about people with terrible illness somehow being treated more humanely in earlier times, and to fantasies that the human condition can be improved by turning back the clock. His stories are reminders of the dangers of nostalgia, and both his commentary and his tone are an enlightening reminder about the virtues of technology. Much maligned high-tech is in fact progress; if romantic notions of an incorrectly imagined "humane" past are imposed on reality, unnecessary heartbreak will be the result.

Before the advent of modern radiation and chemotherapy, in all its gross imperfection, people with leukemia *always died* of it. If they were lucky, they had the companionship of decent people like Dr. Moloney, and the solace of a spiritual life—assets still available to anyone who can find them—but their dying was physically ugly and unenlightening. They were not part of the continuum of cure that is the subject of this book. They were stricken; that was all.

Facing patients' deaths is a problem for the doctor, Rappeport says, if he doesn't have hope for the future. At the same time, he says, "one deals with death by not turning away from the person who's dying," or from the patient's family. He also says that from the moment he knows someone has relapsed, he considers him dead. The fact that he doesn't act on that knowledge—that he keeps trying for the patient—is one thing for which Rappeport praises himself.

He says this at seven o'clock on an October evening in 1989, as he walks along a hospital corridor, on his way to see fifteen-year-old Rich Frisbee. Rich had a transplant the previous January, and relapsed six months later. The news came after a bone marrow aspiration, done at a regular posttransplant checkup, showed leukemic cells. Rappeport told Rich's mother over the phone, and the Frisbees returned to Connecticut from a Cape Cod vacation. The family had longed to go, although Christine Frisbee, worried about the distance it would put between her son and his doctor, had anguished over the wisdom of leaving.

As soon as they returned, in July, Rich started receiving aggressive chemotherapy, aimed at gaining a remission. His family hoped a second transplant would be possible. It would be hard, Christine knew, to achieve a remission; it was hard the first time, the previous December. Then, as she waited, day after day, to see if Rich's fevers would abate, his coughing stop, the bone marrow tests come back with a reduced number of leukemic cells—all necessary if he was to be eligible for a transplant—she said, "I sit here and think, How could this have happened?" And her knitting—navy blue, with fine stitches on a circular needle—sat untouched, with only a few rows finished.

"The hardest call," Christine said when Rich relapsed, "is going to be deciding when to stop the prodding and poking, to take him home for the end, if that's what is to be." Because his leukemia is a combined type, he needs, again, two combinations and courses of drugs—"protocols" Christine calls them, the hospital terminology her own now. And of course, she mentions, the chemotherapy will further reduce his immunity, still radically diminished from the bone marrow transplant that took place only a few months ago. She says her family is okay. Her other four children are fine. Her husband Rick is taking it hard, of course.

"But Rich is doing well," she says—"doing well" is also hospitalese, two words that carry with them the silent connotation "in context"—and if Rick is doing well, then so is she. "It's a roller coaster," she says, using a phrase mothers in her situation say over and over again. And now, using her high intelligence and accustomed competence and the medical knowledge she's gained the hard way, she tries to figure out whether to take the very slight and surely painful chance Rich has been offered—"one in a million," Christine defines the odds—or to take him home to die. She no longer wears the rings she wore six months ago, and her nails are now short; everything has to be constantly washed and kept clean to protect Rich. Nothing else about Christine's appearance has changed, however.

She is slim and small-boned, a blond, beautifully dressed woman, and she is notably down-to-earth. Her husband works on Wall Street. He is a trader for Drexel Burnham, a company recently the subject of scandal and soon, in the midst of the Frisbees' worst trouble, to go abruptly bankrupt, putting all their employees, including Rick, out of work. Through all of this, Chris stays near Rich. She learns the location of every coffee maker, and how to get from one part of the hospital to another through the basement. She makes friends with nurses and doctors and ward clerks. She is gracious. Unfailingly, she asks me about my family— about my children and about Roberta's experience. After Rich relapses, she starts smoking, lighting up with the nurses, and with Rappeport.

In October, Rich is still at Yale–New Haven Hospital, on the pediatric floor where he has already spent months of his life. He does not seem like a child now, though. Tall, thin, and bald, he asks an adult's questions, and knowing what's coming for him, he calls his doctor by his first name. He and Rappeport talk in a small conference room that, at the moment, is serving as Rich's dining hall; a cardboard tray of teenager's carryout sits on the table in front of him. He cries, acknowledging the fact that the leukemia has come back. Still, he wants to talk, wants to understand. Can anything be learned from my relapse? Will people ever know what causes leukemia? Could it be genetic? Could it be environmental? Could it be a combination? Could there be something in the water, for example, and some people are more susceptible to it?

Rappeport asks if Rich has any ideas. "It sounds like you're thinking about it."

"I wouldn't mind knowing," Rich says. "Joel, do you know more than you did ten years ago?"

"More than five."

"How do you know when you know?"

"You know," says Rappeport. "You make observations, you report them." He gives an instance of medical progress made through scientific method: In 1948 someone made an observation about acute leukemia—up until then there had never been a remission—that led to methotrexate, a chemotherapeutic agent Rich knows well. "When I was in medical school," Rappeport goes on, "people didn't live more than two weeks, or four weeks."

"Do you think," says Rich, "that someone will be able to come up with a medicine that will put everyone in remission?"

"Not for every leukemia."

"Am I ALL or AML?"

"A little of both." Rich suffers from a bi-phenotypical leukemia, meaning, explains Rappeport, that the markers on Rich's cells indicated two kinds of leukemia. That made his leukemia difficult to diagnose precisely, and it made it—and makes it now—difficult to treat.

"Is either easier to cure?" asks Rich. "Which cancer shows up in me? Is it one cell?"

"One cell has a little of both; it can't make up its mind. And," Rappeport says, "any ideas would be gratefully appreciated."

Rich is determined to live until his birthday and until Christmas, but he dies early in December. After he dies, Christine comes back to the hospital—over and over again, at all times of the day—to visit and to plan a memorial for her son. At his funeral, she reads a poem she'd written the previous summer, "when I realized Rich wasn't going to make it," Chris says. It's a prayer, really, and her voice is gentle. "Will you smile down on me, Rich," she says, "and help me to laugh?"

A few weeks before, sitting outside a sedated Rich's room, she'd used almost the same words to Rappeport. She does not leave her post; she is with her child until the end she knows is coming. She puts down her magazine and stands up. "When this is over, Joel, will you make me laugh? When I come by your office to say hello, will you say something funny, to make me laugh?"

TWO

≈≈≈≈≈

The Biggest
Obstacle

When black moods descend on Rappeport, his warmth disappears, and the misery he shares every day is reflected back. He holds his lips tightly together. He becomes arrogant, brusquely delivering conventional and absolute judgments about everything. Because Rappeport is an actual human being, not an artifact called *doctor*, there are multiple reasons for the flaws in his personality and the difficulties in his life. But where his effort to overcome fatal disease with bone marrow transplantation is concerned, one complication, above everything else, frustrates and worries him: GVH.

Graft-versus-host disease is one definition of Rappeport's career. GVH, secondary to bone marrow transplantation and virtually unknown outside it, has been the greatest barrier between him and his goal. It is a complicated immunological disorder, the result of lymphocytes in the donor marrow attacking the recipient's cells. That is, the donor marrow (the graft), with its immune system still operating, perceives the recipient (the host) as foreign, and attacks the host because its nature is to attack all foreign substances. GVH is common, but the percentage of people it afflicts is dependent on many complicated variables. The older someone is, the more likely that he or she will get GVH. The greater the genetic similarity between the donor and the recipient, the less likely the patient is to suffer from GVH. This is true especially, but not exclusively, of similarity at the identified antigens of the HLA locus, because the HLA locus includes not only major histocompatible differences, which are known, but also many *unknown* minor histocompatible antigens. Therefore, matching at the major HLA locus, critical as it is, does not provide insurance against GVH, indicating that other genetic matching must be involved. Because Wesley Fairfield is an identical twin, he was essentially protected from GVH, although even that is not absolute; a very mild form of what appears to be GVH sometimes appears in identical twins. GVH is on the lips of everyone involved in bone marrow transplants, but familiarity does not indicate full knowledge, let alone mastery.

There are two basic types of GVH, chronic and acute. Chronic, in this context, means of late onset, first occurring as much as a year after the transplant. The other broad category is acute GVH, defined as that which strikes within the first one hundred days after the donor marrow is infused. The severity of either form varies greatly, ranging from a mild rash to fatal destruction of vital organs. One can have acute *and* chronic GVH.

One of Rappeport's earliest patients, who received her transplant in 1973, at the beginning of Rappeport's career, had one of the first diagnosed cases of chronic GVH. "My skin was so bad," she says, "I walked bent, like an old woman. My skin split open and bled." Before the transplant, "I was pretty and healthy." She was twenty-four, with a two-year-old son. "I had pretty skin, nice hair. I probably never will have hair now." In the hospital, "I used to get upset when a social worker came into my room and asked, 'How's your sex life?' I knew it was to get me talking, but it was a stupid question. My sex life was lousy, but I was in pain from my head to my feet. I just thought it was a stupid question." Her husband left her. Her illness may not have destroyed her marriage, she says. "I can't say it was that, with the way things are today. But I haven't met anyone since."

At grand rounds (a formal educational lecture for the hospital's medical staff), Rappeport uses pictures of her to illustrate GVH at its worst. The photographs are anonymous, not revealing her face. The slides, projected on a screen in a darkened amphitheater, show her straight back, nipped-in waist, long legs, and the skin, brown and red and angry. Rappeport, singling out the most striking patches with his pointer, describes it as looking like a third-degree burn. The woman herself says she did a lot for research. There were all the drugs Rappeport used on her, trying substance after substance in hope of a cure. And, "They used to come in and take pictures of me naked. I'd tell Rappeport, '*Playboy* would pay me for this.' "

She praises Rappeport. He is a "fantastic doctor. When I was in isolation—and I was in isolation for four months—he'd call at one or two in the morning to see how I was doing. In the end," she says, "it's worth it—just to see my son grow up." But she's angry. She talks with fury about a collection agency that's after her for medical bills. "I'll pay, but I just can't understand it. Fifty-eight dollars just to walk in the door. I was there fifteen minutes, they drew a little blood—$800." Her graft-versus-host disease resolved itself, but she talks of the attempts at cure. They took place over many years, but she speaks with a clipped and forceful immediacy. Some of the efforts were desperate; many of them were experimental. "I was a guinea pig," she says. "None of it was Rappeport's fault. But I think maybe it does a number on him. He has aged, he looks like he's tired out. He's never said it to me, but I think he would like to see more progress with GVH. We used to be real good friends in the beginning. I sensed a big change after a year, when somebody died of pneumonia. I thought that took a lot out of him, that he pulled away, then."

Rappeport appears to love many of his patients, but he almost never says so. His affection shows in the calm seriousness of his voice or face, or in an admiring story. It is sometimes evident in a gesture: in order to move closer to a woman on an examining table, he moves her shoes out of the way, picking up and placing them with a respect worthy of the glass slipper.

When I asked him which of his patients he loved, he said, "Peter Lariviere would have to be at the top of any list."

Lariviere says of Rappeport, "I thought he could do any-thing." Nevertheless, he wishes he could be his own doctor. "Any patient knows his own body best." Lariviere suffers from chronic graft-versus-host disease. The acute form attacked him in 1981, while he was still in the hospital undergoing the transplant, and he has been afflicted with the chronic form ever since. He says he'd never do it again, and would advise someone else to do so only if the person had a good match.

At sixteen Lariviere was stricken with acute lymphocytic leukemia (ALL). ALL is the most common cancer in children and, in the United States, the second leading cause of death in children under fifteen. Even at the time of Peter's diagnosis, most children with ALL could be successfully treated with chemotherapy. Peter, however, had a subtype—T-cell ALL—that makes up about a fifth of all ALL cases and for which bone marrow transplantation was then almost certainly the *only* cure. (Now, however, many doctors recommend chemotherapy alone—without a bone marrow transplant—as curative treatment for T-cell ALL.) Without a transplant, Peter would have died before he was eighteen. He did not realize it then, however, and for a long while afterward—a year after the transplant—he didn't know what leukemia was. "I thought it was something that would put me in a wheelchair, like muscular dystrophy."

Now, he's angry at other people's misconceptions. "I get so mad when I tell people I had leukemia and I'm better, and they say, 'Oh, good, you're in remission.' I'm not just in remission—I don't have it anymore." He hates it just as much, however, when his trouble is minimized. "On TV shows they show somebody having a transplant and walking out fine, a week later, from the hospital." He has suffered from the complications of his transplant ever since it took place. "I had so many things wrong with me, I don't even remember—I don't want to remember."

The two-month period of transplantation wasn't so bad—he remembers the chemotherapy he'd gone through earlier as a lot worse. It's the years of illness since. He almost always has a cold. Because of GVH he is immunodeficient and has had pneumonia at least five times. He cannot remember exactly how many times because he has had several different kinds, sometimes with one following another. He has suffered a stroke, is still weak on his right side, and has a slight speech impediment. His hearing in both ears is impaired. His vision is bad; he cannot read many pages without his eyes hurting, and bright sunlight blinds him. When he stands outside, looking at the plot of land he plans to cultivate, talking about the vegetables he'll grow, and the greater scale on which he plans to grow them, he not only wears a hat with a visor but also shades his eyes with his hand.

He is subject to a sudden and uncontrollable need to urinate, as a result of what Rappeport categorizes as "extraordinary" hemorrhagic cystitis, a reaction to the drug cyclophosphamide, standard treatment for a transplant. When cyclophosphamide is administered, a catheter is customarily inserted in the bladder, to make sure the urine, now containing a highly toxic drug, gets flushed out, or as Rappeport always and obscurely puts it to patients, "to make sure it's going the same way you are." Normally, once the catheter's inserted it stays in place for the necessary days. Peter's urinary tract was so inflamed that the catheter kept popping out; during one evening, six had to be inserted, each time making him scream with pain. At least once, he had to be anesthetized. His teeth deteriorated—GVH gave him dry mouth, in addition to dry eye—and they are now all capped. When he grins (which he does often, frequently with his teeth clenched), they seem large in proportion to the rest of his face. He is very thin. His blond hair is sparse. Some areas of his skin are pale, others mottled, some streaked with scars. Graft-versus-host disease has either caused these maladies or exacerbated them.

Treatment for GVH, itself a side effect of bone marrow transplantation, has caused these side effects. When he was eighteen—two years after the transplant—he went to the hospital with stomach bleeding so profuse that he needed seven units of blood. Doctors treated the ulcer responsible for the hemorrhage by pouring ice water into a tube that went from his mouth to his stomach. Prednisone, an anti-inflammatory drug prescribed for GVH, caused the ulcer. (During his transplant Peter was given the then-standard prophylactic treatment for GVH—methotrexate. After he developed GVH, he was prescribed azathioprine and prednisone.) The steroid should have been taken with an antacid, but Peter says no one told him to do so. Brian Smith says use of an antacid may not really help anyway.

In the beginning, when Peter first had GVH, it was "just tightness of the skin. My skin was like plastic. It was taut, and if I got cut or something, it wouldn't come together, wouldn't heal back up. It was like slicing something that was very tight. And just a little scrape would hurt."

Later, over a period of years, the other manifestations of the disease showed themselves, but when he was in the hospital for the transplant, it was his skin that was chiefly afflicted. The outer layer peeled off in sheets, and skin problems have plagued him in the years since. He had massive diarrhea only during that hospitalization, though. His mother remembers a nurse counting seventeen bedpans she'd carried from his room "on just one shift. I was scared. You get scared, when you see something like that." And although Ernie Lariviere, Peter's father, says of course he would advise a young person to have a bone marrow transplant, he'd never undergo it himself.

At bone marrow transplant rounds—a weekly staff meeting where the circuit is verbal rather than physical—nurses, doctors, a nutritionist, a social worker, and a physical therapist sit at a table in the unit's conference room, the door between them and the actual patients shut. Rappeport asks me whether Peter would undergo another transplant if he had it to do all over again. Hearing a reiteration of Peter's opinion, "only if the match is a good one," Smith and Rappeport and one other doctor—the three present with long experience with GVH, both in the laboratory and at the bedside—bow their heads. They know GVH seems to work against leukemia, mitigating against relapse. But they also have seen it, many times, running its unrestrained course, killing people or ending, sometimes with disability, only after years of misery. When a fellow asks why a patient's possible GVH should be tested and treated, why not let it run its course, and perhaps work against leukemia, Rappeport sits the young doctor down for a long talk. "We're *afraid* of GVH," he explains.

Peter Lariviere says he is bitter only over the loss of his friends. "People I knew from second grade never came to visit, never wrote," when he was in the hospital. "I guess that's kids. But family sticks with you. I didn't want the community to raise money, that kind of thing. I didn't want to owe anybody. I fought with Dr. Rappeport every year, to take me off immunoglobulin, because I didn't want to be dependent. I wanted to be independent."

Brian Smith explains that, in fact, patients are better off if they are "independent" in this way. One needs the antibodies that B cells (precursors of immunoglobulin-producing plasma cells)— triggered by T lymphocytes—provide, through a complex process involving additional cells called monocyte-macrophages. The interaction between the different types of blood cells is critical, because a person may have the necessary blood components, but "if the cells aren't talking to one another," says Smith, "you're not going to generate antibody.

"If you are totally unable to make antibodies, or get replacement antibodies, then you can get fatal infections." And a partial, inadequate supply of antibodies results in chronic, low-grade infections. "Often you get pulmonary infections over and over again;

you get lung damage, and some of those people eventually die from that—or, nowadays, come to a lung transplant."

None of this need happen today, because immunoglobulin, gamma globulin—a blood product distilled from donated plasma— replaces the necessary antibodies. (Intravenous gamma globulin was not available when Peter Lariviere first got sick, however.) "We can get away with replacement," Smith says, but "it's not perfect. In a way it's like being a diabetic." Insulin replacement works, but not perfectly. "We still aren't able to give you insulin in exactly the same way that your body would normally make it, and so diabetics tend to get a variety of complications over time. There are some kinds of conditions in which we can basically replace the missing product perfectly well. If you don't make thyroid hormone—and after bone marrow transplant and radiation therapy a certain number of folks become hypothyroid—we can give you thyroid hormone once a day and basically return you to normalcy.

"But with antibodies it's somewhere in between" the efficacy of insulin and that of thyroid hormone. Transfused immunoglobulin, "other people's antibodies, don't necessarily include antibodies in sufficient amounts to deal with every infection you might come up against. It's not quite the same thing that your body does. Your body makes a very specific, very high-affinity, highly effective antibody when it sees a new infection. Replacement antibodies don't really do that. All you have is whatever's in the general pool. So it's not perfect replacement. It's possible that with this replacement, thirty-five or forty years down the line—maybe because they still don't have the body's normal antibody response—people are going to get into trouble. We have no reason to think that is necessarily true, but we worry about it." Ultimately, says Smith, the aim is to goad the body into producing its own antibody adequately, so the patient can "throw the crutches away."

Gamma globulin is also an example Smith cites when he talks about medical progress. It reduces infections and also reduces the incidence of GVH. Gamma globulin and ganciclovir, he says, cure CMV pneumonia. Since CMV pneumonia and GVH are among the biggest killers of people who need bone marrow transplants, gamma globulin and ganciclovir are perfect examples of the "very small changes" that add up to progress over the years.

"Now," says Peter Lariviere, "I'm all cured and I don't owe anybody, except my family. And Dr. Rappeport took me as a son.

I'll tell you, he knew every trick in the book to get me to do things. I never knew how bad it was; that's how I got through it. And you have your own mental power that heals you. The mind's a great healer. So's Dr. Rappeport. My mother says God never gives you anything you can't handle. But I blame Him. Why me? I never did anything wrong.

"Dr. Rappeport's a total doctor, that's about it. But he's also compassionate. He kind of knows what the patient's going through. He's tough with what they have to do, and he's compassionate when something goes wrong."

At the agricultural high school he attended after the transplant, Peter did make a couple of friends; the class president was his date for the senior prom, and later, because of her contact with Peter, became a nurse. But he is still isolated from people his own age. When, after eight years of illness, he was finally able to work—at a farm and market stand near his house—he was grateful for the companionship of a coworker also in her twenties. He lives with his parents and his two youngest brothers. Ernie Lariviere is by far Peter's closest friend. He takes him camping and golfing and will drive him anywhere.

When Peter was in the hospital, unsure if he'd survive, his father told him that if he got out he'd take him to see the Grand Canyon. Later, he did so, driving from Massachusetts. On a telephone lineman's salary, with a family of twelve to support, he gives himself to Peter over and over again. "My father is my backbone," Peter says. "He's my idol." Peter lists the presents he bought his mother for her birthday, describing each with love and pride. His nieces and nephews visit constantly. "Kids are what I love best," he says.

On a visit to New Haven to see Rappeport, he stops for a long time outside the room of a little boy undergoing an autologous transplant (one in which the patient's own marrow is used) after treatment for retinoblastoma.

Retinoblastoma is a rare disease of great scientific interest, because the normal function of the genes responsible for it is negative: they are supposed to curb cellular growth, and when they fail to do so, tumors form. It may be that this mechanism comes into play in other cancers as well, and because the genes in retinoblastoma have been identified and mapped—they're on a part of chromosome 13, a subdivision of the ql4 band called the *Rb-1* locus—

they can be cloned and studied, thus leading to a greater understanding of cancer's dynamic.

The disease can be either hereditary or sporadic, the first meaning it runs in families, and the second meaning it's caused exclusively by outside influences—that is, by anything, such as infection or toxic chemicals, not native to the organism. In addition, an error in replication can cause the faulty gene. In that case, the problem isn't with the sperm or egg, and therefore isn't hereditary. Instead, a genetic copying error—anytime after the egg and sperm are formed—causes the defect. Since one gene in a pair will compensate for another's dysfunction, however, both must be knocked out for disease to occur. In the sporadic, nonfamilial form, outside influences—"accidents," as Rappeport puts it—completely account for the disease. In the familial type, an inborn mutation in the *Rb-1* locus precedes the external assault. The little boy Peter visits probably has the hereditary form of retinoblastoma, because he's had the disease in both eyes, indicating that four genes (a pair for each eye) are nonfunctional; it's unlikely that accidents—either in replication or outside influences—could alone account for such damage. Instead, he's almost certainly the victim of a combination of bad luck—first the congenital blow, then another from outside sources—that gave him tumors in both eyes.[1]

This "double hit" frequently comes up in Rappeport's diagnoses, but for this patient Rappeport is serving less as a detective than usual. The child had already been diagnosed and treated when he came to Rappeport, and the purpose of the transplant is a straightforward and relatively simple rescue mission. Some of the boy's marrow was removed and frozen before he received what Rappeport refers to as "a *lot* of chemotherapy," treatment so aggressive that it destroyed his bone marrow—not itself diseased—and he's now gotten the stored marrow back.

Before chemotherapy the child's eyes were irradiated, but that treatment failed to eradicate the cancer growing behind them, and so he had surgery, entailing the removal of both eyes. He was learning Braille in nursery school before the cancer came back, his grandmother says. Despite the conditions of his life, the little boy plays happily in his room and except for his bald head looks normal; the prostheses in his eye sockets look like the real thing. His grandparents, talking to Peter, are proud of the little boy's accomplishments and pleased with his progress. Like Lariviere, they are smiling, obviously glad to have their grandson alive, and hopeful for him.

Peter does not refer to the fact that he is sterile. He does not talk about whether or not he hopes to marry. His parents worry about how to help him to be more independent, how to keep him from becoming depressed, how to find the right occupation for their bright son. "Dr. Rappeport said if Peter wanted to be a doctor, he'd help him," Ernie Lariviere says. But Peter does not talk much about the future.

Peter Lariviere's mother and father characterize their relationship with Rappeport as "all business." "We didn't bother him with trivial things," Louise Lariviere says. "He was always in deep thought," says Ernie Lariviere. "You'd be talking to him and you'd know that he was almost thinking about a patient he'd just seen, and trying to solve *his* problem. But," he says, "I don't think I'd want any other doctor but him taking care of Peter."

Peter's cataracts were not a result of GVH; they came from the radiation he received. His memory of that experience is vivid; he says radiation tastes the way bleach smells. In 1981, when he had his transplant, radiation as preparation for bone marrow transplantation was given in one huge dose, rather than being divided into several sessions over a few days, as it was by Wesley Fairfield's time. And high, concentrated doses of radiation, it is now known, are likely to cause cataracts. Before surgery for them, Peter needed thick glasses, "Coke bottles" he and his family call them. He hated being seen in them. During the same period, in order to protect himself from infection when out in public, he had to wear surgical gloves and a mask. People thought he had something contagious, and moved away from him as he waited at elevators and at the window of the newborn nursery, where his father took him, on visits to the hospital, in order to cheer him up.

He was emaciated, too, then—he weighed 89 pounds, down from 128 before he got sick; he weighs 117 now—and he was bald. "When he got out of the hospital, Peter looked like my grandfather," his sister Laurie says. People still stare at him. "It's his hair," Laurie says. "He looks normal other than that."

Gary Lariviere, the donor for Peter's transplant, says, "You go with him anywhere and feel the stares; it's his build." But it's not only Peter's thinness. "You can see in his face something's wrong, something's different." Gary was twenty-eight when he was a donor, and he had never heard of a bone marrow transplant. Like

Scott Fairfield, he had heard the word "leukemia," and that was about it. "I knew that leukemia equaled bad blood—bad white cells. But I figured they'd irradiate Peter, put in mine, and he would be normal. It still hasn't done it. The doctors didn't say Peter would be back to his old physical self, but I thought it would have done more for him. The family's athletic. The other kids are well coordinated. Peter's coordination isn't even close to what it used to be." Gary never questioned serving as the donor. "It was for Peter. And hey, if it was me . . ." and he alludes to a bond that didn't exist before the transplant, giving a physical example: Peter has sinus problems he hadn't developed until then, and Gary has sinus trouble. Peter probably acquired this problem from his brother, as it would have been part of the donor's immune system. Gary concedes that Peter's getting better, but "I think when I see him that graft-versus-host is still there."

Peter thinks it is; he points to "my year-round tan," the brown patches on his hands and forearms—graft-versus-host disease starts on the torso and moves toward the extremities—but Rappeport says he thinks the disease has burned itself out now. The effects are still there, though, evident in the respiratory infections that debilitate and worry Peter every winter, and the vision problems that for years prevented him from getting his driver's license, the necessary key to liberty and independence in the rural Massachusetts area in which he lives. His family's house, at the end of a long, tree-lined lane that runs from the road, has a pond behind it, and enough land and trees around it so that no other buildings, except Peter's greenhouse, are visible from it. With Rappeport in Connecticut now, Peter sometimes goes to a local doctor in his town, or to the community hospital, but they haven't always been willing to cope with him. Sometimes when he goes in with a complaint, he says, they look at his chart and close it. They send him home with an over-the-counter cold remedy, useless against the serious coughs and fevers that have brought him. His sister Laurie shrugs. "A decongestant can't hurt you, right?" When Peter was in the hospital in Boston, his chart was so full the covers of the binder bent outward. Close to home, the doctors haven't always dared to touch him.

Laurie remembers sitting in a car outside a local doctor's office the day Peter found out he had leukemia. The beginning of the story is just like the Fairfields': Peter had had a sore throat and a headache, but it was January—"the flu season," his mother says—

and she didn't make anything of it. But then, he looked awfully pale, and she took him to the doctor.

Peter says it was a nurse, a woman who had worked at Boston's Dana Farber Cancer Institute, who was suspicious first. They drew blood and the next day called: Peter and his parents should come in right away. Laurie says that when Peter came out again, he said, "I want to die." Peter, however, says he said the opposite: "I don't want to die." And now he says, only half-jokingly, that if he gets really sick, and his mother takes him to the local hospital instead of to Rappeport, and he dies as a result, he'll come back to haunt her. When I quote this to Rappeport, he groans. "That's all she needs; she's already consumed by guilt." And he's right. Like every patient's mother, Louise Lariviere worries over and over and over again about why Peter got sick. She says she blames herself. She thinks up possibility after possibility, none of them based on objective fact. "Maybe God thought Peter could take it. Maybe He chooses the strongest. Maybe I should have done something different." She can't think what. But "A mother always blames herself," her daughter Laurie says.

At the end of a long day visiting Rappeport at the hospital, Peter Lariviere goes home with him. He's been invited for dinner and to spend the night, but he gets there later than planned. As Rappeport's clearing his desk, getting ready to leave the office, he opens a letter and discovers the donor for a recently transplanted patient has hepatitis. On the day of the marrow harvest, there was an accident; Rappeport's hand slipped, and he squirted part of a syringe of marrow in his own face. Now he learns he's been exposed to hepatitis. He swears as he reads the piece of paper, but he doesn't, at first, explain what's happened. "He told us he didn't use drugs!" he says of the donor. "He swore he didn't!" Rappeport gets up and looks at his shelves, pulls out a heavy book, looks something up, puts it back. "I'm just going to stop up at the floor."

At the nursing station, he talks to a fellow, turning his body so he can't be overheard. He makes a phone call, the fellow looks something up, Rappeport sends Peter to the cafeteria to wait for him. A half hour later, he appears and explains: He was looking for an antidote, and the fellow gave him an injection to prevent hepatitis. He's still worried, however, about the damage to which the recipient's been exposed.

At home, Rappeport eats dinner and goes into the living room, where he collapses in front of the television set, one hand on his dog, the other holding a cigarette. His eighteen-year-old daughter walks in from a shopping expedition and whips the short leather skirt she's just bought out of a shopping bag. "Want to see it on me, Dad?"

"Not now, Amy."

In the kitchen Linda Rappeport sits talking to Peter, asking him about his greenhouses, about the plants he grows. Peter describes them with great interest and pride. He's said that in school he loved growing things, liked science and math, but didn't like high school English. He did love *A Separate Peace*. He read that novel three times. His problem with literature, he says, is that he didn't understand the symbols, although he was the only one in his class who figured out the riddle in *Oedipus Rex*. He knew that no matter how many legs the creature was supposed to have, no matter what kind of a shadow it cast, it was a man.

Peter came as a patient to see Rappeport, but he spent the day as an observer, looking through microscopes, talking to other patients, listening to debates outside patient rooms and to discussions in front of computers that convey patient lab data—the latest blood counts and drug levels—at the touch of a key. He's seen the crowded visiting room, heard the phones ringing and the beepers paging.

His meeting that morning with Rappeport was a reunion. They hadn't seen each other for a couple of years and each of them—Peter, especially—was forthright about his wish to see the other again. The meeting was classically masculine in its casualness: a handshake, Rappeport busy and solemn, Peter with a quick joke. All through the day, into the evening and the next morning too, he's delighted to see the Rappeport he knows. After breakfast on the second day of his visit, right before he leaves, he asks Rappeport if he thinks he did the right thing, choosing to have the transplant. His parents had said that at sixteen he was old enough to make the decision. Does Rappeport think he made the right one? Rappeport states the options, cites the statistics. Though they add up to the fact that a transplant was Peter's only real chance, he stops short of giving a conclusion. Peter crows with laughter. "He never gives you a straight answer! Never!"

And afterward, reflecting on the view he's gained as a visitor and a medical insider, rather than as a patient, he doesn't talk about his suffering, but states his understanding—typically, for Peter, full of compassion: "It's hard for the doctors, too."

*   *   *

When talking about specific patients, Rappeport is given to
speaking pessimistically, with what seems to be a superstitious
caution. In one way or another, things won't work out. He seems
sure of that. An insurance company will refuse to pay or will delay
so long the patient will be too sick to cure. A patient is too sick to
undergo a transplant; it probably won't be possible to induce the
requisite degree of health and really be able to help him. Another
is dehydrated; yet another is hospitalized with a respiratory infection; it's questionable whether the first can be persuaded to drink
enough, doubtful if a relatively new drug will work against a previously incurable pneumonia. Rappeport's actions and the events
that follow belie his moroseness. Phone negotiations with the insurance company and completion of their cumbrous paperwork end
in a commitment to pay the bills without long delays. Constant
care, twice- and thrice-daily evaluations result in a remission of
disease, allowing a transplant. Long talks with the dehydrated patient and his family persuade them to force liquids. The patient
with pneumonia is well and on his way home.

Technology may or may not instigate cure, but it does effect
it. Six months earlier, Rappeport had taken the train into New
York—a city he hates to visit, because its scale frightens him—to
confer with representatives of a pharmaceutical company that man-
ufactures a new kind of gamma globulin. This is a drug potentially
useful for anyone with a diminished immune system, a category
into which GVH patients, like Peter Lariviere, fall. Rappeport is
always dubious about the unproven, and sure there is no magic
bullet. Still, he can cite the first comprehensive study on GVH—in
1960, by a man named Billingham, done on chickens[2]—and it is
Rappeport who reels off every drug ever used on a patient, before
or after a transplant, to avoid GVH or ameliorate its effects, he who
alludes to floundering in search of a cure, but who remembers every
attempt and its result. It is Rappeport who lists, over and over
again, in every forum, the benefits of bone marrow transplantation
versus the risk from an imperfectly matched donor, and who directs
the implementation of new attempts to overcome that gap.

At a tony week-long summer meeting of basic scientists, held
on the campus of a Vermont prep school, Rappeport gives a talk,
and moderates a panel, on bone marrow transplantation and gene
transfer. In July 1989 this is the hottest of topics, and Rappeport is
what he calls "extraordinarily" nervous about the quality of his

presentation. Afterward, he says he was the only one there, out of about 150 participants, without his own laboratory. Brian Smith says Rappeport did fine, the meeting went well, everyone had a good time. At an international gathering of scientists working at the cutting edge, Rappeport has, unsurprisingly, held his own. But the insecurity he regularly admits to and his friends refer to offhandedly, is in evidence: a photograph of the thirty or so speakers standing in the sun shows everyone but Rappeport in shirtsleeves. He's wearing a windbreaker and is the only unsmiling person in the picture.

Lucy Cabral sits on a hospital-issue plastic chair, her daughter Carmen on the table waiting for Rappeport, and talks about the reality of full-blown chronic graft-versus-host disease. Carmen, twenty-four, usually comes alone from Bermuda for her checkups, but she has had a bad scare on this trip: her cornea has torn, she doesn't know how badly—she wears a patch over one eye—and she's sent for her mother to join her. Lucy reports that she dropped everything and hopped a plane right away. She is incisive in her description of the effect of GVH. "It is terrible for us. Terrible for Carmen, of course, and for all of us." Her speech, and her daughter's, have a slight West Indian lilt and the edge of an English accent. She shows snapshots of their house—stucco, with a winding driveway and a travel folder's sunset and background foliage—and tells Rappeport she wishes he'd come for a visit. When Rappeport protests over a present Carmen has brought him, her mother quiets him: "She wants to do it, Dr. Rappeport, because she loves you so much."

Carmen is beautiful. "Gorgeous!" Brian Smith says of her. She has large dark-blue eyes and a straight nose, perfectly proportioned lips and even white teeth. She is slim, with high full breasts, small waist, narrow hips, long legs. Her long dark hair, however, is actually a wig. And her skin, from head to toe, is a mottled and shiny brown, except for the places it has torn and is a bloody red. Even the clinic staff were shocked when they first saw her. "Was she burned? What happened to her?" But they are tactful, and do not show their feelings. Rappeport says that Peter Lariviere used to look every bit as bad.

A nurse says that when Carmen visits, and they take walks together, or go out to lunch, people stop and stare at her. She says only the cure of GVH will make Carmen feel better and that she is isolated with her disease. According to the nurse, her family can't really understand Carmen's distress, because they are just glad she's alive. But Lucy Cabral seems to understand very well. Bermuda is a small place, and Carmen is the only one there with her problem. Lucy also talks about people staring. And Carmen, on a previous visit, has said there's no point trying to cover her skin with makeup, because everyone she sees knows how she really looks. On this visit, though, Carmen is happier than she's been before. Despite her worry about her eye and the diarrhea she's been having and the weight she's been losing—perhaps because of a thyroid problem, possibly acquired from Lucy, her donor—the GVH, present since shortly after her 1985 transplant, seems to be diminishing. The redness in her skin is an improvement, a sign of normalcy breaking through. Her toes are pink, and the same color is beginning to show on her legs. She has been taking a drug, effective against the leprous lesions of Hansen's disease but new for GVH, that is apparently working. Brian Smith saw a report of the drug that piqued his interest, and Rappeport has decided to try it on patients with GVH.

Carmen is wearing a hospital gown, and when Rappeport tells her she looks great in blue, she laughs. There is the usual crowd in the tiny examining room: Rappeport, Carmen, Carmen's mother, a nurse, and a resident. Often, even more people are present when Rappeport sees a patient. He gives the resident a short course on GVH, with Carmen as the object lesson. She never had kidney involvement. That is worthy of note both because it is usual— GVH generally doesn't affect the kidneys—and because it is the rare organ in Carmen's body that GVH has not afflicted. Rappeport points to places on Carmen's neck where there had been "big ulcers—they were holes," and the nurse and Lucy Cabral concur. Things are better—Carmen says they are, and everyone else agrees—since she has been taking the drug.

Once GVH has manifested itself, it disappears again in only three ways: by running its course, by the use of immunosuppressants—usually cyclosporine, azathioprine, or prednisone—given after the transplant, or by the death of the patient. Rappeport says cyclosporine, an immunosuppressant discovered in 1972, has had a major impact in preventing graft rejection in solid organ transplants, but overall hasn't been effective in bone marrow transplantation. "It's a tough drug to use," he says, referring to side effects, but even aside from that he's not sure there have been gains from it.

It has been effective in acute severe GVH in HLA-matched and partially matched transplants. As it's currently being used—in conjunction with methotrexate—it halves the incidence of that form of the disease. It is not clear, though, that it helps with chronic GVH. And so, "It may be apples and oranges," he says. "You may pay the piper later in terms of chronic GVH."

In those people for whom GVH is a predictable danger, therefore, Rappeport and Smith concentrate on prevention. In the past, they've worked with monoclonal antibodies produced to work against the T cells, whose presence in the marrow is presumed to cause graft-versus-host disease. "There's a price for everything, though," says Rappeport. Just as chemotherapy before a transplant and steroids used on GVH after it cause problems, T-cell depletion on the marrow itself—after it's taken from the donor and before it's transfused into the recipient—also can cause damage. The T cells he's reducing in order to ameliorate GVH are the same ones that are necessary to the normal immune system. They're the cells AIDS patients lack. With a weak immune system, the patient will be subject to every kind of infection; with no immune system, he'll eventually die of an infection. A too-vigilant donor immune system, on the other hand, will trigger GVH, maiming and perhaps killing the recipient.

You can reduce T cells through the use of monoclonal antibodies. But what's a monoclonal antibody? "Say you wanted to make an antibody against Rappeport," says Rappeport. "Take Rappeport cells and inject them as a foreign agent into some other species" such as a rabbit. "We would put in some things to make the immune system greater; we might inject the rabbit again ten weeks later. Then a few weeks later, we'd test the animal, bleed the animal, and we'd have anti-Rappeport. You can't just inject the cells into another rabbit, because that rabbit might not respond with the same kind of antibodies. He may make a different anti-Rappeport antibody. Basically a monoclonal antibody immortalizes the particular animal antibody—in this case, mice—immortalizes the mouse antibody you want. So let's say we want anti-Rappeport right eye. We will inject Rappeport into some mice. We will then screen the antibodies these mice make, and we will find one, two, out of thousands of spleen cells, that make anti–right eye.

"We then take the B cells from those mice—the B cells that make the desired antibody—and immortalize them by fusing them with a mouse multiple myeloma cell. Now, a multiple myeloma is a malignancy of the B cell, or the plasma cell, and that is one way to immortalize the antibody-producing cell. Then, you can keep it in dishes and the mouse can die and that cell will keep growing in a dish forever. It's a tremendously labor-intensive project when one's searching for a specific antibody, but once one gets it, one can then grow these things up in vats. There are qualities of the antibody that have to be satisfied. It has to be an antibody that recognizes the cell you want it to recognize. It has to be an antibody that doesn't recognize the cell that you don't want it to—you don't want it to kill off the bone marrow stem cells. It has to be capable of binding with the protein complement because complement and antibody together are what will lyse the cells, disintegrate the cells, the T cells causing graft-versus-host disease.

"However, a cell is not too dissimilar from the whole organism. If I start to beat you over the head with a baseball bat, what are you going to do? You go like this." Rappeport shields his head with his arms. "Well, a cell does the same thing. It tries to protect itself, and so the markers on the cell that are being recognized by the antibody start internalizing; the membrane turns on itself and pulls these things in, and now the cell can't be attacked any longer; it's protecting itself. So the particular antibody we've used has a poison attached to the back of it. The marker turns into the cell, the antibody goes with the marker, and on the tail end of the antibody is this poison that will poison the cell once it's in the cell—it's the Trojan horse approach, if you will."

It's a technology that hasn't been all that effective, Rappeport says. And it isn't that interesting to do, says Smith. And the pharmaceutical companies they've dealt with have given them headaches; there've been difficult people at one place, and unreliable batches of the antibody have come from another. They're ready to try out another method, one that predates monoclonal antibodies, when the appropriate patient presents herself.

She does so in the form of a three-month-old baby, suffering from osteopetrosis, in which the bones' cavities—the place where the marrow belongs—fill instead with bone. Without a bone marrow transplant, the baby will die. It would take at least three months to find an unrelated donor, and in that time the baby, probably already blind, will go deaf; bone is growing into the skull cavities through which ocular and auditory nerves grow. The middle-aged parents, both in their second marriage, the mother childless up to now, have told Rappeport they are willing to raise a blind child but worry about caring for one who is deaf as well. Nevertheless, they have decided to go forward with the only hope they have for her. This "marble bone disease" is genetic, but the baby has a related, unafflicted donor: her grown half sister, whose marrow is an imperfect match. To avoid the GVH that would certainly follow the infusion of untreated, poorly matched marrow into the patient, Rappeport and Smith have decided to investigate— through applications to this baby—one of the two methods of T-cell depletion they've been considering.

Starting at 7:30 on a February morning Rappeport harvests the marrow with a throng of assistants—house officers and nurses who have asked to be there—and by 9:30 Brian Smith is driving to New York's Memorial Sloan-Kettering Hospital, where there's a laboratory that specializes in the technology. Steve Ginsberg, a hematology fellow, sits beside Smith in the passenger seat, a Styrofoam container holding two bags of marrow, and two test tubes of it, packed in ice on his lap. I'm in the back seat, taking notes as Smith explains to me the laboratory technique we're going to see, and also answers my questions about osteopetrosis and about the comparative results of no treatment, matched donor transplants, and haploidentical, or half, matches in bone marrow transplantation. He and Steve Ginsberg also talk about alternative routes from and in New York and all three of us express enthusiasm for our chosen road, the Wilbur Cross Parkway, which avoids Bridgeport, over Route 95, which is far less scenic.

We also debate the abusive behavior of a patient's relative, which we've all recently experienced, along with Rappeport and the entire nursing staff. What's the provocation for her hostility, and how should we respond to it? Should we talk back to her? If so, what do we say? Is the distress of the family a good enough excuse for attacking the innocent—us? Do members of a patient's family— even fairly distant ones, as this woman is—merit the same restraint and forbearance that we all agree the actual sufferer deserves? We reach no conclusion. Although each of us has imagined a confrontation in which we score a pure moral and practical victory against the offensive relative, none of us knows what we'd do in an actual battle, or even what we ought to do.

Bone marrow transplantation works in osteopetrosis, Smith says, because in the disease the deficiency in bone modeling originates in the marrow. In marble bone disease, the more descriptive name for osteopetrosis, osteo*b*lasts (one set of cells necessary for bone formation) perform their function, laying down bone, but another cell type (osteoclasts) fails to remove the old bone, as it is their function to do. No one knows where osteoblasts originate, but osteoclasts derive in an unknown manner from monocytes, a blood cell derived from the marrow stem cell necessary for hematopoietic development. Therefore, the osteoclast is a cell derived from bone marrow, and via bone marrow transplantation osteoclasts, necessary to preserve the bone marrow space, can be restored to the patient who has osteopetrosis.

A description of marble bone disease doesn't make it seem like a blood disorder. The result of the osteoclast's mal- or nonfunction is that the victim's system suffers a layering of bone in the marrow cavities that eventually, Smith tells me, "squeezes out bone marrow, which goes to the spleen, and fills in holes in the skull that nerves come out of, squashing eye nerves, hearing nerves, the nerves she needs in order to eat." Untreated, the baby will die before she's a year and a half old. Even if the graft takes, damage may be irretrievable; nerves that are destroyed completely don't regenerate. She may be left retarded, as well as blind and deaf.

An imperfectly matched relative isn't optimal, and T-cell depletion has its problems, but that combination is the child's best option. Therefore, Smith and Rappeport decide on Sloan-Kettering's technology. Smith is going to New York to see for himself how it's done. If he and Rappeport decide on the method, he'll be able to replicate it in New Haven.

It's a variation on the technique Rappeport described as "the Trojan horse approach." The goal is the same: to remove the cells likely to cause GVH, while leaving behind those necessary for a graft. The difference is that technicians, rather than using poisons to kill the T cells, physically separate and then remove them from the marrow that's to be infused into the patient. This is done with two substances, both of which sound very low-tech. It's the way their actions are used that reveals an underlying knowledge of molecular biology.

First, soybean lectins, which bind to T and B cells, are used to attract unwelcome cells, and that part of the marrow is put aside. B cells are removed not because of GVH but because lymphoma, a B-cell disease, occurs more frequently in people who have had an HLA-mismatched transplant than in the rest of the population. Most T-cell depletion methods don't try to diminish B cells too, but Smith says it's probably a good idea to try doing so. He says also that the discovery that depleting the marrow of B cells reduced the incidence of lymphomas was made retrospectively and serendipitously. "That's the way science works."

After this initial depletion, red blood cells—erythrocytes—from sheep, are added to the remaining marrow. They bind to human T cells. The sheep erythrocytes surround T cells in formations that look like the petals of a flower—thus the procedure is called rosetting—and since these clusters are now denser than the rest of the marrow, they fall to the bottom. The marrow is spun in a centrifuge, after which the division is obvious: the bottom portion of the fluid is red, the top is clear.

Smith explains the problem this technique is to solve. In order to avoid both GVH and graft rejection, the fraction of the marrow with T cells will be irradiated so they can't proliferate. They'll give this part to the baby shortly before she receives the T-cell-depleted marrow. On the one hand, the host immune system seems to attack incoming stem cells if no T cells are present, so that no graft takes place, but on the other hand T cells can't be allowed to proliferate, since they seem to be GVH's instigator. Thus, the idea behind the method is to strike an illusory balance. The irradiated T cells are to act as decoys, living long enough to trick the immune system into allowing the stems cells to establish themselves, but dying before they can trigger GVH. Essentially, it's a bluff.

This lectin and rosetting protocol is described on an instruction sheet as "Human Soybean Agglutination (SBA) Sheep Red Blood Cells (SRBC); Preparation for Transplantation by Removal of Alloreactive T Lymphocytes." Smith says it is "straight out of the Amazon." And he likens all efforts at T-cell depletion to those at gene transfer, the technique in which a normal gene replaces the abnormal one that causes a specific disease. With every T-cell-depletion method, he says, "Every basic scientist in the world said it would work, because in the lab everything does. Whereas in people it screws up."

Smith constantly ridicules living in the abstract while ignoring the concrete. When a pharmaceutical company tries to hire him, he goes for an interview. He has no intention of taking the job, but he tries to persuade the people with whom he's meeting that at least one doctor in their company should spend some time with patients—one day a week, say—so they can really understand the effect of their drugs on actual people. Smith sighs at the naiveté of a biomedical think tank. They ought to come up against an actual sick person too. He himself spends about a quarter of his time with patients, and insists he's a doctor rather than a basic scientist, and it is true, as Rappeport points out, that Smith always seems concerned about people. He never agrees to a simplistic formulation of human nature, whether it's applied to an individual personality or a major social issue. "It's more complicated than that" is his constant response. "And so," he says, again likening still-theoretical gene transfer to the mixed and incomplete success of T-cell depletion, "nobody knows what will happen. And if gene transfer does work, it will be in ways one hundred percent different from what everyone thinks now."

The scientists running the rosetting laboratory at Sloan-Kettering are welcoming and interested, both in their work and in the patients they hope will benefit from it. They talk about "washing" the marrow—mixing it with solutions to purify it of substances added as part of the separation process—and about rosetting the cells, about how their chief encourages contributions for equipment, such as the elaborate microscope Smith admires, about delays in operating room schedules that mean marrow will be harvested hours later than they expected, keeping them at work far into the night. Nancy Collins, the head of the laboratory, says the hours are long anyway.

"The unrelateds," she says, referring to marrow from donors unrelated to the recipients, "don't even come in until 5:30," and the many hours of T-cell depletion follow that. She and Smith agree enthusiastically that the way in which the bags of marrow are hung under the sterile hood is ingenious. "That's what advances science," says Collins, "the little things." Smith admires a plastic tray, called a "cell farm," that sorts cells. Collins and the technicians who work with her reassure Smith that they'll keep some marrow in reserve, in case the first try at achieving a graft doesn't take.

When it comes time to pack the marrow for its trip back to New Haven, Collins stuffs gauze between the plastic bags and the ice; direct contact will kill the cells. All along, she has asked questions about the recipient, and responded with anecdotes about other people for whom the process has been done. There's no reason to think she's ever seen any of them, but it's evident that they're all real and important to her. She tells Smith she'll call him the next day to see how everything went.

The actual procedure has been complicated and tedious, and it's clear that success is impressively dependent on people being careful with a long series of mechanical steps. A technician is constantly tending the marrow, watching it, tapping it, shaking it, moving it from container to container, machine to machine. She shakes bags of plasma, pipettes some off without disturbing the agglutinate on the bottom, waits just the right amount of time between one step and the next. The process is outlined in thirty-seven points that include not only technical directives but also instructions such as "screw the cap back on." The last item is "Have bagels and eggs and go to sleep."

At 8:30, Smith calls Rappeport, tells him what's happened so far, and then leaves with the Styrofoam container and Xeroxed instructions. The whole procedure has taken nine hours, faster than Smith expected, and at 10:30 he's back in his own lab to check the marrow—what Collins refers to as "the graft"—for clumps. At 11:15, with Ginsberg helping him spin, check, and treat the marrow, he says that the clumps are out and that he's resuspended it "in a nice solution a baby like that can take. Without messing up its lungs." At 11:30 he and Ginsberg walk over to the bone marrow transplant unit, Ginsberg with one syringe of marrow, Smith with another: the presumably stem-cell-rich component and the substance with the inactivated T cells that's to be used for the trick maneuver.

The unit's lights are turned low for the night. It's dark in the patients' rooms, and the area right outside them is lighted only enough so nurses and doctors can read charts, check equipment, make sure of dosages. The baby is connected to machines that monitor her blood pressure and heart rate. She's getting oxygen through a hatbox-like clear plastic device placed over her head, and like all bone marrow transplant patients, she gets blood products and nutrition intravenously. She sleeps, sedated in preparation for the transplant. She is round-faced, with a spray of light hair. She still looks normal. Toys sit beside her in her crib.

Rappeport joins Smith, who, working from outside the plastic curtain, through its rubber gloves, infuses the marrow. They talk about other patients and about the baby's condition. They agree that the separate infusion and the injection of ATG (antithymocyte globulin)—a serum used to induce immunosuppression, in this case used on the theory it will help the baby accept the graft—is "hocus-pocus," but Sloan-Kettering's methodology mandates the use of both, and they follow the protocol.

Everyone's tired. Steve Ginsburg has collapsed onto a chair at the nursing station. Smith, sitting on a stool outside the baby's plastic curtain, keeping an eye on her, tells Rappeport, who's standing by doing the same thing, about the day in New York. Nancy Collins is "very nice," he says. His tone is gentle.

Smith and Rappeport's friendship is mutually protective. Each frets over the other's missed opportunities, and worries when he thinks the other is unhappy. They have separate careers—Smith, especially, is involved in science and medicine not directly related to bone marrow transplantation—and different family lives (Smith's a bachelor), but their shared life is critical to both of them. They have the same intertwined ethical and scientific understanding. They have had much of the same experience, and have much the same view of people, although Smith, who is the more articulate of the two, is more analytical and far more likely to discuss somebody's personality at length. He can, therefore, seem warmer, more involved with people than Rappeport, but it is the latter who never wants to acknowledge the end of a relationship, who broods, sometimes obsessively, over what he sees as exclusions, particularly from a patient's care, and who, when he's gruff or rude to someone, is hurt and mystified at the person later resenting him. Smith is much more objective about other people's trouble, much more calm and consistently kind-voiced in response to problems people bring him, but he has an unpublished telephone number. It's Rappeport whom patients call at home, and it's he who listens to distraught relatives in the middle of the night.

Neither Rappeport nor anyone else can predict with certainty which of his patients will die, which will be healthy, and which will be afflicted with severe GVH. It is for sure, however, that none of them would have a chance without a doctor willing to take a frightening risk. Because Rappeport is an exceptionally well-informed practicing specialist working on medicine's cutting edge, his patients are dependent on the soldering of his ethics to his knowledge. It is he who must decide, for each person who comes to him, if he has a chance worth offering. In this context, GVH is not only a problem but a standard. Since Rappeport knows his patients will die without him and must be sure that healthy life is worth attaining, it is the middle ground—pain and ill health—he has to evaluate. It's there that the question of whether the cure justifies the suffering is at its most grindingly acute.

Rappeport was prepared to spend the night at the hospital if

Smith had taken longer in New York, or if the baby had needed to be watched longer. But at 1 A.M., after the transplant, he walks to his car, talking to Smith about problems he foresees with the nursing staff. He frets about the system, wishes he'd be allowed to participate more in solving the nurses' problems, fears a disaster (it never materializes), and drives home.

Three months later, the baby's still in the hospital, and sicker. At six months, she no longer looks normal. Her face is swollen and her cheeks are so huge she seems misshapen. Rappeport denies that perception. She's fat, he says, not swollen. Though she receives all her nutrition intravenously, he says she's been "eating too much." A nurse agrees, but she's anxious about the baby, who she says is "awfully fussy." She clucks to the baby, pats her, and working through the plastic curtain's gloves, tries to get a blood pressure. She can't get an accurate reading, and paces between the baby's room and the nursing station, where she picks up the phone, calling to get a more usable cuff; the baby's arm is too plump for the infant's size they have on hand and too small for the other obtainable size. The nurse is agitated; she snaps at the other nurses and addresses her worry, partly as an appeal and mostly as a monologue, to Rappeport, who sits on a swivel chair talking to the house officer currently assigned to the unit.

The baby's skin is bright red. Since there's no sure evidence a graft has taken effect, it's unlikely she has graft-versus-host disease, but if she does, it would be a great worry. They have to know for sure. First, Rappeport will check the HLA typing of the baby's lymphocytes to see if they are the same as the donor's. If they are, and not the same as the baby's before transplantation, then GVH is a possibility, and Rappeport will perform a skin biopsy to see if she has it. If she does, she's in trouble, because, with its immunosuppressive quality, GVH is particularly dangerous in a haploidentical match; its presence is likely to reduce the chances of the graft taking a firm and permanent hold. The result, of course, would be lethal.

Hematology fellows draw blood from the baby and then, using recombinant DNA techniques, "amplify" her DNA—that is, increase the amount so they can read it. They then look to see if it matches those areas of her donor's HLA type known to be different from hers at the time of the transplant. The comparison shows that the baby is producing cells she and her half sister didn't previously share. This means there's at least a partial graft. (GVH would prove this too, of course. "You have to have a graft to have GVH," as Brian Smith puts it.) The baby's doing better clinically, too, and at the beginning of July, Rappeport's planning to send her home, to see "if the graft's enough in terms of disease." The disease in question is not GVH, but osteopetrosis.

"The reason for this," says Brian Smith, referring to the question of quantifying the transplant's success, "is that in genetic disease a 'partial' graft may be plenty—the host cells are abnormal but not malignant. They can stay around and not get the patient in trouble. The trick is to get enough of the *donor* cells to stay around also, to provide enough osteoclasts to reverse the disease. For reasons we don't always understand, however, when both host and donor cells are present together the host cells usually eventually fully take over."

Meanwhile, the baby's skin rashes still come and go, but a skin biopsy's shown no evidence of GVH. She's been in the hospital for nearly all of her seven months, much of the time on the bone marrow transplant unit, some of it in intensive care. At least once, it looked as if she would die. Her mental status is unknown, but it is clear that she has "deficits," as the concerned nurse puts it. The baby has not yet sat up, turned over, or fed herself. Her parents, screaming in anger, have refused the CAT scan that can determine brain damage. They say that first they have to know whether she'll live, but Rappeport says he'll have to insist on the test, that they have to find out if the child's retarded, and he needs a baseline in order to monitor her progress.

This isn't the worst possible outcome for a patient needing a bone marrow transplant. All the parents I talked to for this book were grateful if their child was alive, regardless of the problems, sometimes acute, disturbing, and permanent, with which they were left. Those whose children died continued to mourn, no matter how long ago their loss had been.

In bone marrow transplantation, a terrible trade-off always exists: The person may be cured, but he may die. If he does, his dying is likely to be more painful and protracted than it would be with less aggressive treatment. If he lives, he may be left disabled, perhaps disastrously so. The baby with osteopetrosis is a demonstration of the promise of the research potential of bone marrow transplantation and of its therapeutic scope. No matter what her fate, the mechanisms of osteopetrosis, of half-grafts, of T-cell depletion will be at least a little better known. For her and her family, the outcome may also be a study in bone marrow transplantation's current shortcomings.

The baby died when less than a year old of respiratory illness, without signs of meaningful neurological or motor development but with some engraftment apparent. The mother told a house officer that she didn't want to talk to Rappeport again, that doing so would only remind her of hard, sad times. The remark was reminiscent of one Martha Fairfield made two years after Wesley's transplant, in incomparably happier circumstances. "There are some people you like a lot," she said, speaking of Rappeport, "and hope you'll never see again."

Whatever bone marrow transplantation's inadequacies, however, it isn't necessarily a failure. This infant's parents decided to take their only chance for what was likely to be their only child. Rappeport says that parents of children with malignancies "fight for every day" of life. My middle-aged sister accepted the probability, and then the reality, of severe—though ultimately controlled—graft-versus-host disease. She lived through weeks of pneumonia so severe that she became unconscious. Having recovered from that, she suffered the completely unexpected complication of progressive, radiation-induced paralysis. It was a fate she was willing to accept. She would still be able to think and to see people, and, she said, "relationships are everything." She would suffer anything, would put up with whatever quality of life she could get, in order to have a chance at maintaining them. Peter Lariviere has seemed on occasion to live in suspended animation, sometimes, after winter upon winter of pain and sickness, unable to rouse himself from depression, at other times full of hope. Year by year he is able to do more. And he's alive.

THREE

≈≈≈≈≈

Blood Itself

*R*icky Stott died, at seventeen, in 1976. "He lived two days less than two years after the transplant," his mother Sis says. She did not know death was imminent—indeed, never believed he would die—but it was she who found him gone, in his bed in the morning. The cause of his death was graft-versus-host disease. At the time, almost nothing was known about GVH, but a good deal was known about aplastic anemia, the illness with which Rick, then fifteen, had been stricken two summers earlier.

In this devastating disease, there is no malignancy. In most patients with aplastic anemia it is lack of cells, rather than mal-formed, dysfunctional ones, that causes the lethal problem. In the early seventies Rappeport wanted to narrow, and thus begin to answer, the questions his biggest problems posed. The first bone marrow transplant in which he'd participated, as a medical student, was on a patient who had acute monocytic leukemia. But once he "had a choice," as he puts it, he decided to begin, "predominantly," with transplants for people suffering from aplastic anemia. The reason was scientific. He could best study bone marrow trans-plant's effectiveness in a disease where he could eliminate the possibility that the invasion of destructive cells—leukemic cells—was the cause of death.

In working against aplastic anemia, he still had the major worries of graft rejection and GVH, but in the absence of leukemia, recurrent malignancy—a relapse of cancer—was impossible. With aplastic anemia, therefore, Rappeport had better reason to hope he could cure his patients and simultaneously reduce the variables—at a time when *all* bone marrow transplants were experimental. Aplastic anemia can be worse than leukemia, Rappeport says, because "it can kill you quick—within days."

The Stotts came to Rappeport toward the beginning of his career; Ricky was his twentieth bone marrow transplant patient. Rappeport was critically and permanently important to the Stotts, and their impact on him has to have been at least as great. His obligation to patients can't vary according to their characters, but his feelings must.

Sis Stott does not have to say she believes that life has a purpose and that people are good, because she so clearly represents these hopes as fact. She talks with a plainspoken certainty, rather than force, and her philosophy is present in everything she says, both in the meaning of her words and in her manner. The mother of four, she has lost her two sons and her husband. The boys—Carl and Richard—died in the midseventies, within two years of each other. She says her husband, also called Carl, never recovered from the blow. "It's the hardest thing that can ever happen to a parent, really," she says, "the hardest thing." She is not simply repeating the obvious. Out of her own experience, and her examination of her husband's, she is stating her knowledgeable and considered assessment of the truth. Sitting at her kitchen table in a Philadelphia suburb, her oldest child Kathy with her, her youngest child Donna joining us at the end, she tells me the stories I've come to hear—of Rick's illness, Carl's fatal accident, her family's relationship with Rappeport.

After her sons died, she did bear it, did go on. She had one daughter in her early twenties, another in her early teens. "You look at the other people," says Sis. "I looked at Kathy. Even more so, I looked at Donna. She went from a home of four children [two girls and two boys], in no time at all, she was here by herself. I'd look at her—she was thirteen, fourteen years old—and I'd think, What's going on in her mind? And you think"—Sis characteristically switches away from the first person—"how can you sit back and feel sorry for yourself? How can you not try to deal with this? Other people are dealing with it. Kathy had just had a baby—a new granddaughter. There's new life. And this is what you try to concentrate on more than the loss. Because it would just—it's—it would overpower you. It really would. I don't think you'd go on, if that's all you did."

In July of 1974 "Rick got a real bad nosebleed," says Sis. "We didn't think too much about it, because our other children had had nosebleeds." But then, "He started getting real listless and just not himself, but really didn't give any great indications of being sick. But just because of your mother instinct, I decided to take him to the family doctor—Dr. Connors—and he decided to do blood work on him."

Kathy says Rick had been bruising. "Symmetrically. One here, and one here, one here, and one here." She uses her own body as an example, placing her hands on her shoulders, on her hips. Rappeport says the only significance of the symmetry is as an indication the bruises weren't the result of obvious external injuries. Kathy was a first-year nursing student when Rick got sick, and remembers her mother calling her at school, saying Rick was sleeping a lot, that he just wasn't himself.

"And when the blood work was done," Sis says, "we got a phone call at midnight from our family doctor saying that Rick's blood was very low, and he wanted us to call Dr. Day, who was a hematologist at a big hospital, Temple Hospital, in Philadelphia. We set up an appointment with him, and took Rick down there. And Dr. Day called us that very night, and told us that Rick had a 90 percent chance of dying. That his platelet count was 5,000. And I said, 'Well, what's a normal count?' And he said, '250,000.' And he said he could really hemorrhage at any time." In fact, Rappeport says, people with aplastic anemia make normal platelets. Smith points out that this means normal in terms of *function*; people with aplastic anemia have abnormally few platelets. Rappeport says that eventually (sometimes very quickly) the level of production drops as far as it's going to, and stabilizes. Some people, he says, walk around for years with platelet counts of 5,000.

Dr. Day told the Stotts to bring Rick in for a bone marrow aspiration. That was followed by a bone marrow biopsy, in which a plug of marrow is extracted and examined. This is necessary for a definitive diagnosis of aplastic anemia, where the absence of cells, rather than their abnormality, has to be determined.

Rick would almost certainly die, said Dr. Day, unless he could have a bone marrow transplant. And that depended on whether there was a match within the family and whether there was an available bed in one of the three hospitals in the country—in Seattle, Baltimore, and Boston—that in 1974 offered bone marrow transplants. Dr. Day preferred Boston. It was farther from Philadelphia than Baltimore was, but Sis remembers Dr. Day saying that the program in Boston was innovative, and the results good. "And because of Dr. Rappeport. Joel," says Sis. "Dr. Day said there were very, very good doctors up there." But room for only one bone marrow transplant patient at a time.

Dr. Day says now that he did not consider giving Rick androgens. More than a decade earlier Dr. Louis Diamond had noticed that his male aplastic patients sometimes recovered spontaneously at puberty, "when they started to shave," Rappeport says. Diamond's observation has held up, and male hormones are still used to treat aplastic anemia. But, Day says, he doesn't think they work very well. Smith concurs, saying they work only in mild aplastic anemia, and not in the severe form Ricky had. Day did try corticosteroids, used to repress the immune system in order to allow marrow to regenerate.

He didn't try ATS (for antithymocyte serum) or ATG (for antithymocyte globulin)—animal-derived immunosuppressants. Even if he had wanted to, they might not have been available; because they are a biological product, supply is erratic—often limited or nonexistent. And they work erratically, as well. Some animals produce more efficacious serum than others; one now-dead horse called Caesar (Rappeport says horses are usually used because they are big animals) cured 75 percent of the patients on whom his ATS was used, but ATS sometimes does nothing at all or causes a prohibitively severe allergic reaction. ATS and ATG function by suppressing the overactive immune system often inherent in aplastic anemia, thus allowing blood's regeneration. Rappeport used ATS on Ricky—to prevent graft rejection—as part of the preparation for his transplant. It was known at the time that ATS helped prevent graft rejection, Rappeport says, but what he learned from this protocol, used also on a number of other patients, "contributed to the concept that in some cases aplastic anemia itself is autoimmune." He's happy at this advance in knowledge, and proud of his part in it.[1]

Today, another group of biological substances is in the forefront of hematological discussion and practice. Growth factors designed to enhance or instigate specific cellular growth are moving from experimental to commonplace use, and their variety is expanding. G-CSF and GM-CSF (for granulocyte colony stimulating factor and granulocyte macrophage colony stimulating factor) are now licensed drugs that can temporarily raise white cell counts and thus fight infection. Other growth factors affect other relatively mature cells, and some are being developed to encourage the more primitive cells that produce functioning end products.

Rappeport says he probably wouldn't use growth factors on a patient such as Ricky Stott. Ricky's youth and the fact that he had a donor mandated the use of a bone marrow transplant, and Rappeport is still disinclined to use growth factors in his transplant patients. But for a patient without a donor on whom ATS had failed, or for someone who was infected and needed a temporary boost in white counts, he'd use GM-CSF.

There are risks to the growth factors. With these new substances, Rappeport is moving with his customary caution and skepticism, but their use and variety are expanding. In some bone marrow transplant centers their use reduces the length of the hospital stay, and as their effectiveness and limitations are better defined, they'll have wider application. But bone marrow transplantation, with or without growth factors, is still the best chance at cure for someone with severe aplastic anemia, as it was in Ricky Stott's time.

Then Dr. Day took two critically important actions. The first was restraint in the use of blood products, because when aplastic anemia patients are transfused before a transplant—especially if the blood used is the future donor's—they are likely to reject the graft. Dr. Day gave only washed red cells—blood from which the white cells, the immunological component, had been removed.

His second lifesaving action was to get in touch with Rappeport. "I called Joel soon after the boy came," he said. Bone marrow transplantation was young, but Day knew Rappeport had experience in it, especially with aplastic anemia. "Joel's data has held up, too," he says. "There wasn't much time lost; we made the decision fast."

"I remember Dr. Day not giving a whole lot of hope, really," Kathy says. "You know, it was just pretty cut and dried, this is what he has and the chances are slim. There were very big ifs—if there's a donor in your family, if the hospital can accommodate you. He gave you the impression you needed a miracle to get to the point where you could have the transplant in the first place."

"You didn't have to know much," says Sis, "to know that it was very, very serious and that the only thing you could do was pray and hope. Pray that you could get Rick to Boston and that maybe something could be done. I can remember being in that room in Dr. Day's office. And him sitting there. Telling us to try not to let Rick get hurt, because if he started to bleed, he would bleed to death, and I thought my husband was going to pass out. He said, 'Don't be telling me this about my child.' He just couldn't believe that this could be happening to one of his children. I thought he was going to get up and punch Dr. Day. And this was not him. It was just so shocking to him, to be told that his child might die." On the drive home, Sis says, she thought her husband was going to pull the steering wheel out of the car.

Carl Stott, Sr., died in 1989, but he left behind a description of the first weeks of Rick's illness. Sis thinks her husband's purpose in writing it was to release some of the feelings he found it so difficult to talk about. The four and a half lined yellow sheets are filled with his emotions, but Mr. Stott never mentions them directly. Instead, his unfinished record is one of observation and information and action, one staggering detail after another packed onto the page just as they are in life when one is dealing with horrific illness and cutting-edge attempts at cure. Carl Stott, Jr., was found to be a match for Rick, a bed was available in Boston, and the family packed up and left Pennsylvania, traveling in the motor home in which they would stay—Sis throughout, and the rest of the family when they could—during Rick's three-and-a-half-month-long hospitalization. It had been only a couple of weeks since the diagnosis.

Aug 11 1974
    My wife and I, and family Kathy 19, Donna 13, Carl Jr. 17 met Dr. Joel Rappeport for the first time. He is a handsome *gentle* man 6' tall, lean and has a very warm and personable smile. Also for the first time we found out what aplastic anemia is, it is the failure of the Bone Marrow to make Red Blood cells, Platelets, and white cells, in other words, he said, Rick's Blood factory is on strike. He also told us that repeated exposure to "DDT", Benzene products, anything in aerosol spray cans, some forms of narcotics [Rappeport says he never said narcotics. Mr. Stott is probably referring to some

antibiotics], and certain antibodies can cause this disease. Dr. also had us bring Rick's medical and pharmaceutical records for the preceeding ten yrs., and asked us if we knew if Ricky had been in contact with any of these things in an effort to determine the cause. In Ricky's case the cause is still unknown. Dr. Rappeport then started talking about the cure. . . .

In aplastic anemia, still, the cause is usually idiopathic, or of unknown origin. A few types are hereditary. Because the propellant for aerosol cans is different from what it was in 1974, they are probably no longer the culprit in aplastic anemia, but several chemicals react in the systems of a small number of people (the vast majority of exposed people never get sick) to cause the disease. Rappeport decided on hematology partly because of his early encounter—in 1964, his last year in medical school—with his teacher's aplastic anemia, instigated by the commonly used antibiotic chloramphenicol, "a good drug," he says, although "there have been a lot of successful lawsuits against it."

Rappeport does not romanticize his decision for hematology, however. Its intellectual pull was strong, in contrast to a number of other specialties, many of which, at one time or another, he's categorized to me as boring. The overwhelming arrogance of particular doctors and his own pride discouraged him from others; an early inclination toward orthopedic surgery disappeared when residents, entertaining women in their bedrooms, ordered him to bring meals and leave them outside their doors.

But there was altruism also, the wish—with Rappeport's personality, the ardent desire—to try to help those who, without him, would be lost. Of course, he responds, too, to goodness in other people, and with the Stotts there was a natural attraction that must have contributed to Rappeport's tirelessness. Sis tells of Rappeport coming to the hospital at one in the morning to reassure her, at a time when Ricky, undergoing preparation for the transplant, ran high fevers.

For a patient with aplastic anemia, Rappeport's preparative regimen for a transplant does *not* include irradiation, because there is no need to kill malignant cells, as there is in leukemia.[2] The drugs Ricky and other people with aplastic anemia receive are given to suppress the immune system so that they can accept their donors' marrow. Immunosuppressive therapy is now given, too, to reduce graft-versus-host disease, which in aplastic anemia not only is as dangerous as in any other bone marrow transplant but also has no potential usefulness. Without leukemia, there can be no antileukemic effect.

If, in aplastic anemia, the donor and recipient are identical twins, in half the cases there is no need for any preparative therapy. (In the other half, Rappeport says, there is pretransplant suppression of immunity because there are indications of autoimmune disease.) Today, Rappeport talks about "just dumping in the marrow" in such an instance and, when faced with it, does just that, transplanting a ten-year-old girl with her sister's marrow and discharging her from the hospital within days. As soon as the new marrow has begun to engraft, her health is better than before she got sick; there have been no radiation and chemotherapy to reduce her immunity, and she's in no danger from GVH. The case seems simple, but Rappeport sees the little girls as a scientific opportunity. "One needs to think about these rare situations—identical twins being rare. Not that many identical twins have been done." Smith adds that identical twins "are the baseline control of what happens if you're getting back totally normal bone marrow that's also totally identical to you." In this example, it's a look into a possible future. If donor and recipient cells could be made to interact as if totally compatible, and if the original disease could be pinpointed and destroyed without damage to the rest of the body, the degree of sickness and danger and attendant emotional distress intrinsic to nearly all bone marrow transplants today wouldn't exist. The financial expense would be greatly diminished, too.

Ricky Stott's transplant (that is, the infusion of Carl's marrow) took place on September 11, 1974. After Ricky was released from the hospital, the Stotts stayed in the Boston area for a time, so that Rappeport could monitor Ricky's health in a more or less normal environment. On December 5, the Stotts returned to Pennsylvania. And on January 5, a Sunday—Sis was at Mass—Carl, Jr., was killed. He was scheduled for early graduation from high school, but because of his brother's illness had not finished some of his assignments. In order to complete a photography project, his father and he set off on a dirt bike, Carl, Sr., driving, Carl, Jr., riding on the back. "He had his helmet on," says Sis. They were up on a hill, "And there's the train there. And the train came around as my husband was coming around a curve." It is one of the very few times in our conversation that Sis's voice weakens. "So," she says, but does not finish her thought. The father survived, the son died.

Rappeport went to the funeral. "He was wonderful to us," Sis says, her voice picking up again.

After Carl's funeral, Ricky got pneumonia. "There were so many people at the funeral," Sis says. "And there was no way that you could have everyone put on masks." The Stotts flew back to Boston, where Rappeport met them at the airport. Sis and Carl, Sr., stayed with the Rappeports. Linda Rappeport—who remembers many nights, during this era, moving her own little girl into her son's room to make room for a sudden guest—waited up for them. The following summer, when Ricky was better, he spent a weekend at the Rappeports' island house in New Hampshire. "So many things that aren't your normal things for a doctor to do," Sis says. "I truly love the man for all the things he did."

For a while after the transplant, Rick was better, although he was brokenhearted over the loss of his brother. They were close, Sis says, "but they were brothers. They bickered." "They were very different," Kathy says. Pictures show Carl with light brown curly hair, wearing glasses and a mortarboard. Ricky, before he was sick, had dark, shoulder-length hair, and brown eyes. They both look self-assured and happy, nice kids. Rick "idolized his brother," Sis says. "He told me, one night when we were talking—after we had gotten over the shock of Carl being killed—'I know one thing, Mom. That Carl was so strong that he put a dent in that train.'" But Ricky just could not accept Carl's death, Kathy says. "That a normal, healthy person, who had saved his life, would die." And Sis says that he "felt so bad that he never got around to formally thanking his brother. And I said, 'Rick, if it were Carl, and you were the donor, would you expect him to come and formally thank you? It's your brother, and you just . . .'" But "even at the funeral, he just couldn't say thank you enough to him. You know, when he was by his casket and everything. And I said, 'He knows. He knew, when he was here.'"

Like his father, Ricky wrote about his experience, hoping the *Reader's Digest* would publish his article. It's written in perfect schoolboy longhand on paper taken from the hospital: "Peter Bent Brigham Hospital" is printed down the side of each sheet, and there's a box in the corner of each page labeled "For Addressograph Plate." The dots over the i's, and the periods, are formed as circles. Rick uses quotation marks frequently, not only to indicate that someone is speaking but, more often and importantly, to emphasize words fraught with meaning: "aplastic anemia." "The doc." His

mother came to see him "every day." The piece is dated "1/25/
75"—twenty days after Carl was killed. Its title is, "Has It All been
Worth It."

> Hi, my name is Richard A. Stott. I'm 15, have brown eyes and
> hair, and weigh about 120 pounds.
> I'm writing to tell you a little about my life, and someone very
> dear to me, my brother. First, I'm the younger son of four children.
> I was born on April 3rd, 1959, attended St. Bede School for seven
> of 8 school years, and now am attending Council Rock High School.
> I enjoy motorcycles, girls, cars, baseball, and am constructing a
> model H.O. railroad.
> My life was abruptly interrupted when in the summer of "74"
> I hadn't been feeling well.

In the next five pages, Rick describes his diagnosis and the transplant, including Carl's experience as a donor.

> Carl was given medicine to relax him and was ready for the opera-
> tion to take the marrow from his hip. It was said that he got up to
> a hundred needles in order to give the marrow. After recovery Carl
> could hardly move he hurt so much. Still he was proud and happy
> that he could have helped me.

At the end of the essay, Rick tells of Carl's death:

> I was working on my trains "on Sunday," January 5th, around
> twelve thirty, two policemen came to the house with My Dad and
> informed us Carl Jr. had been fatally injured by a Penn Central
> freight train. While doing a photography assignment for school.
> "With luck," a priest had been passing by and gave Carl his last rites.
> He's in heaven now, and happy he has to face this world of crime
> and hate no more. Carl did a great thing for me. He gave me his bone
> marrow and saved my life. "I love him for that, I love him also for
> being himself, for giving and taking and acting the way he did for the
> seventeen years he lived." Out of generousity, two weeks before
> Carl was killed, he gave his eyes [that is, he signed an organ-donor
> card]. Now because of him two people are seeing.
> Although my brother's death was tragic to me, my family and
> many others, we cannot let this stop us. We must carry on with our
> lives, with only memories to bear.

The Stotts' trouble was not over. For a while, Ricky was well
enough to return to school, but he was still sick. He drove a car—

"His brother's GTO, a very popular car with young people," Sis says—he saw his girlfriend, he was godfather to Kathy's daughter, but he wasn't well. Ricky had GVH, induced, says Rappeport, by a sunburn. He remembers seeing the sunburn, and he is sure it is that which triggered the GVH. It is because of Ricky Stott's experience that Rappeport now insists his bone marrow transplant patients protect themselves against the sun, but the Stotts have no recollection of the event. They are sure they were not instructed to keep Ricky out of the sun, and they are right. At that time the sun's role in GVH wasn't known. They couldn't have been warned. A year before Ricky's illness, in fact, another of Rappeport's transplant patients spent an unscathed summer as a lifeguard.

Sis does not remember exactly when GVH manifested itself, but she and Kathy both remember what it was like. "It was like his skin didn't fit him anymore," Kathy says. It was so tight, so leatherlike, that it seemed to constrict his ability to eat and to breathe. Sis massaged ointments into his wounds, Kathy helped him to exercise, so that when he got better he would have the full use of his limbs.

In April of 1976 Carl Stott, Sr., suffered a heart attack, and there was talk of selling their house and moving to the shore, where they had another, smaller place and it would be less expensive to live. Rick worried over this possibility, Sis says. "It seemed like he was doing okay. But his attitude wasn't as good as it should have been, I didn't think. It just seemed like he was failing. I don't know if he was just more upset about his dad than he should have been, or whether then he reverted back to thinking of Carl more. But he just became weaker and weaker." It never occurred to his mother and sister that Ricky would die. "It didn't seem God could put him through all this and not have him live," Sis says.

Nevertheless, it is implicit in Sis's entire telling that she blames no one. She never expresses hate or bitterness. Her acknowledgment of loss takes the form of gratitude. Not only Rappeport, she says, but the other doctors and the nurses too were kind beyond any expectations. "We had no family in the area. They were our family." Their neighbors helped. The parents of Rick's girlfriend drove her to Boston so she could visit Ricky. On follow-up visits in Philadelphia, Dr. Day waived his fee. A friend of Kathy's took Ricky for rides; his friends came over to see him. Sis is concerned that I understand how kind people were to her. How wonderful her own family was, how "extremely caring and giving Karen and Rose and Betty," Rick's nurses, were. They all came to visit the Stotts in Philadelphia. How good her neighbors and friends were. "So many people helped," Sis says. "You don't do it alone. There's the big guy up there. And many, many wonderful people."

And Rick was "a wonderful boy. A super boy." He loved the outdoors, he loved getting on his bicycle in the early morning to deliver papers, because he loved the fresh air. Anything he put in the ground grew. In memory of his brother, he planted a twig that is now a birch tree. He had little gardens all over the place. He liked the Carpenters, Donna says, and Kathy adds, "He liked girls." "He used to say when he grew up he'd marry a sturdy wife and have a bunch of girls to do all the work, and one boy, and he'd be the king." "He was a jokester," Sis says. "He'd say he had to tie his shoe, and put a foot on a chair, and then lean down to the foot still on the floor, and tie that shoe." He was generous. "He'd give anyone anything."

It is beyond dispute, because in its essence if not its details it is a completely accurate self-portrait; surely Sis Stott's son was as she describes him.

Ricky died September 9, 1976. Sis called Rappeport in the morning to tell him. Rappeport was as unprepared as the family. GVH was still a new disease, its course unmapped. "He was devastated," Sis says. "Some of the nurses told me."

When I asked Sis for a picture of herself, she sent one that included her husband. It was taken on a cruise to Mexico in 1988, "in happier days," Sis said; Carl, Sr., died not long after their return. In the picture, Carl and Sis are seated behind a glass-laden, lamp-lighted table. They are smiling and bright-eyed, dressed up and carefully groomed. Streamers hang behind them. Carl's arm is around his wife, his hand pressing into her shoulder. Folds of her light blue chiffon dress are visible between his fingers.

Rappeport has not told me how he felt about Ricky Stott, or what he felt when he died. I would be astonished if he did so, though he is a man of such enormous feeling that my mother, even at a time she was completely inundated with the sorrow of my sister's terrible fate, looked at him and said to me, "He's so intense he looks like he's going to explode." And added, "The poor guy."

Rappeport's effort to maintain life in the face of death is a constant. Certainly this wears him down, but it also sustains him. His discomfort comes from other sources, too, particularly from injustices he thinks have been directed against him. He focuses on what he imagines to be his failure to prevent, avert, or deflect them. Most of all, he broods about his move from Boston to New Haven, blaming it on himself, the structure of academic medicine, and the doctors who grabbed power he wanted and deserved.

He seems to have been squeezed out because of what people without much respect for governmental process call "politics," meaning jockeying for position and ruthless power grabs. In academic medicine, antipolitical cynicism ranges from Rappeport's insistence on not dirtying his hands by engaging himself with people he categorizes as "street fighters," to those very people judging a doctor's worth by the quantity (not necessarily quality) of publications and his or her demonstrated ability to bring in money through grants and donations.

Rappeport did not want to leave Boston. Except for four undergraduate years at Yale and a stint in the air force, he had always lived in the Boston area until, when he was nearly fifty, he moved to Connecticut. He believes that the Harvard teaching hospitals are peerless. And because he is affectionate and tenacious, he remains attached to the people and places he's known all his life. Once, I asked him if he missed Boston. "I'm not into change," he said, and then sank into a sad, angry, mostly silent mood that lasted at least for the hours I then spent in his company.

Rappeport is frequently irritable and impatient, and has aggravating oddities. The way he communicates, for example, along with his sense of time, tends to be highly idiosyncratic. When he makes a business call at eight or nine o'clock at night, he's surprised, even indignant, if the other person isn't available, although he resents the telephone's intrusion when somebody else is doing the calling. When he tells a story or gives an explanation, except in a clear teaching situation, he tends to start in midthought, omitting the beginning and leaving the listener with a bewildered sense of having turned on a news broadcast already under way.

He feels he hasn't published as much as doctors in positions like his are expected to, and blames himself for it, but the reason is partly virtuous. It's true Rappeport hates to write, and procrastinates or avoids having to do so, but it's also true that he doesn't stoop to the common practice of putting his name on papers describing research he hasn't been directly involved with, or supervised. Still, the fact that he finds it difficult to delegate does make for inefficiency and frustrates other people.

Nevertheless, as far as I can tell, the issues that provoked Rappeport's job change have nothing to do with either good patient care or the advancement of science. An English doctor who did his training on both sides of the Atlantic told me that in Boston, "politics" are worse than anywhere else, because of the intensity of competition; there the hospitals, crowded against one another, are staffed with the most highly educated, presumably most talented, doctors and scientists in the world, often duplicating programs, usually not sharing information, racing for prizes and prestige. "They didn't pay any attention to Joel," says an old friend and coworker, a doctor and scientist who got the boot from the same crowd. "It was like elephants stepping on an ant." He speaks as if being edged out was inevitable, and long before the New Haven move he had advised Rappeport to leave.

Sis Stott's recollection of Rappeport is correct but incomplete. It omits the creaking and bangs common to the workings and inefficiencies of all businesses, including science and medicine, and the strain and weariness that have accumulated over the years since she knew him. It leaves out the verbal whacks he takes at the people around him: A fellow doctor is stupid, Rappeport tells him in public; a woman present at a staff meeting is unattractive, he says, in front of her, illustrating an anecdote. It would be sentimental to expect Rappeport to be perfect, but it would be equally so to ignore the fact he is not.

Rappeport's stated philosophy of never turning from—let alone against—a dying patient is only partially fulfilled. After a particularly generous-hearted and spunky young woman has relapsed, he avoids her when she comes for a clinic visit. This patient's prognosis was always bad; her widespread disease was not fully in remission at the time of the transplant. Nevertheless, Rappeport was haggard the day he had to tell her the transplant had worked for only a few months. His skin seemed pulled down, loose against the bones of his face, when he came into his office and fell heavily into his chair at the end of the day. Weeks later, when the young woman sits in the clinic, eating carrot sticks while a drug used to slow the growth of her malignant cells drips into a vein, Rappeport busies himself in another part of the big, open chemotherapy room. A fellow puts Rappeport in an office chair and wheels him over to see the patient. The ride's supposed to be a joke. But a social worker reports that the young woman says she feels she's been deserted.

And Rappeport sometimes, without apparent evidence, attributes anger to people in trouble. A young couple come to talk to him about treatment for their little girl, who needs a transplant, but of an exotic type Rappeport isn't equipped to perform. The markers on her leukemic cells show them to be of a special type called CALLA, for common acute lymphatic leukemia antigen.

The little girl is to have an autologous transplant rather than an allogeneic one. That is, some of her own marrow will be taken from her, and then, after she's had intensive chemotherapy and an attempt has been made to purge any remaining leukemic cells from the extracted marrow, it will be transfused back into her. Rappeport points out that this isn't a true transplant, since nothing's being taken from one person to give to another, and so there will be at least one less complication—there won't be GVH—and he also explains the necessity of going elsewhere for the procedure.

Although the type of leukemia is common, the technology is specialized. Only a few places have it; it would be inefficient, simultaneously more expensive and less curative, if it were otherwise. The child should be treated at a medical center with a laboratory specially equipped to do the necessary purging for this particular type of leukemia. In sending these people away, Rappeport is acting in their best interests. He says so.

The man and woman sit and talk for an hour, explaining not only their daughter's physical condition but her emotions and personality. She cries every morning before school, they say. She has been undergoing chemotherapy for years. She is exceptionally bright.

"And now," says Rappeport, "she's special in another way." Yes, the parents say. And they have a younger child, too, a toddler, and the 150-mile commute to the hospital in which their daughter will have to stay is a problem. Rappeport is impatient with that complaint; he says it isn't that far to travel. They ask what this big place is like. Will they actually see the doctor who's expert in CALLA transplants? Rappeport explains, weaving in the reasons he can't do the procedure himself, in this hospital, which they already know and which is close to home. Throughout, the parents have been calm and attentive, polite and straightforward. "We understand," the mother says. "We're reasonable people."

They are, but after they leave Rappeport interprets their visit as a plea. They said they came for information, but in conversation about them he disregards their statement, and focuses only on the fact that he said no to them. His understanding of the situation makes him accusatory. With his face stiff, his voice nasal and cramped, he says that they're very angry at him.

Rappeport's world is a paradoxical scene: suffocating but vital, traditional but groundbreaking, emotional but technical, filled both with petty tasks and with life's most important questions and its biggest issues. His effort for Ricky Stott, and for all his patients, is part of an overall understanding, and of a daily life that always includes the conference room and the laboratory, as well as the bedside. Most basic to his work, and most complicated, is the study of blood itself. Rappeport is most at ease—or anyway, least tense—teaching about that.

Medical students and residents regularly gather in the laboratory for Rappeport's excruciatingly exhaustive, and ritualistic, combination diagnostic and teaching sessions. In diagnosing a patient, in examining bone marrow aspirations and blood smears under the microscope, Rappeport uses an acute eye, an encyclopedic memory, and an alert perceptiveness for physical subtlety to make his evaluation. The length and intensity of his experience have everything to do with his astuteness. Neophytes can't do it—the students and trainees regularly get it wrong. Rappeport sets them straight through the Socratic method.

At the sessions, Rappeport controls a set of microscopes rigged so that four people look at the same slide. Most of the slides are of the bone marrow and "peripheral blood"—blood drawn out to be studied—of people who are currently hospital or clinic patients. The trainees sit at the microscopes, the long work areas in the rest of the room littered with a laboratory's paraphernalia of beakers and bottles, the light from the tall windows filtered through an urban hospital's soot. Rappeport announces it's time for the Four Questions, explaining to the non-Jews present that this refers to the part of the Passover Seder when the youngest person present has to speak.

Rappeport sits at the microscope, genial and relaxed, turning a wheel to change its power, treating the slides with first one drop of oil, then another. These are the stains that make the cells visible, and there's talk of "getting good touch preps"—of readying the samples for examination. He moves the visual fields and the microscope's pointer in order to bring his students closer to the picture that will enlighten them. The more primitive cells can't be seen at all under the microscope. Their progeny indicate their presence;

there can't be a macrophage without a myeloid stem cell, for example. "Move to the left," he says to a student sweating out an answer, referring to the hematopoietic chart on the wall. He means that the young man's mistake is in identifying a cell as more mature than it is, that he should consider stages closer to the stem cell in giving his answer.

Diagrams showing blood's cellular development are omnipresent in hematology laboratories, and in department offices and conference rooms as well. On the left or at the top, depending on the diagram, there's the self-perpetuating pluripotent stem cell, which divides into two other stem cells, the myeloid and the lymphoid, which also subdivide. The lymphoid stem cell separates into two developmental lines, one of which culminates in the B cell, or plasma cell, and the other in the T cell. The myeloid stem cell is much more prolific. According to the hematopoiesis charts, it has twenty-eight descendants leading to six functioning end products that carry oxygen, help clot blood, fight infection, and clean, digest, attract, and sort other cells, in the blood and in other tissues throughout the body.

According to Rappeport, the definition of the cells is nowhere near as precise as their schematic representation suggests. This is, after all, a developmental process. For example, if we fully understood the mechanism of blood cell division, and could see exactly where and how it went wrong in leukemia, cure would follow. But it's hard to know, even in the case of a particular person with "clinical evidence of disease"—with symptoms—exactly where the problem lies.

The names for the stages of cells are artificial; it's really a continuum. Immature white cells are bigger than older ones; the nucleus gets smaller as they mature. A poly (for polymorphonuclear leukocyte, also called a granulocyte or neutrophil) probably can fight bacterial infections from the time it's a myelocyte on, but not before. Again, Rappeport indicates the hematopoiesis chart on, the wall; myelocytes directly precede polys in development. Lymphocytes are a bit smaller than granulocytes, and, unlike them, all look alike, solid and dark. A normal erythrocyte—a red cell—is about the size of the nucleus of a lymphocyte.

The pictures of these cells in textbooks, and on the posters and wall calendars and blood atlases that pharmaceutical companies give to doctors, look terrific, whether they're drawings or tremendously enlarged photographs of the real thing. They're at their most gorgeous in the photographs of Lennart Nilsson.[3] As with his pictures of embryos and fetuses, Nilsson has penetrated life's secrets in order to present us with its mystery. There's a macrophage, its net of tendrils swilling up a noxious invader. There's another one, which Nilsson calls the "armoured tank of the immune system." His astonishing picture makes it look so: a mass of green globules and tendrils, an especially long one projecting like the barrel of a gun. His picture of a thrombocyte shows it among other cells, emphasizing its small size, presenting it as a little ball that, fulfilling its clotting function, adheres within an injury and helps form the plasma's fibrinogen into fibrin, crucial threads in a blood clot. With Nilsson's help, that netting is visible, too. Granulocytes are seen as round, also, but much bigger than thrombocytes and craggier; they're uniformly covered with tendrils. There's a swarm of mature erythrocytes, round red pillows, each discrete, looking smooth and uncomplicated, actually coursing through capillaries. Erythrocytes are round but not globular. They're more or less flat, but biconcave, having a single indentation on each side.

Erythrocytes, filled with hemoglobin—the oxygen-carrying pigment that makes red cells red—have no nucleus. This fact is frequently alluded to indirectly when someone's undergoing a bone marrow transplant, because immature red cells do have a nucleus, and so their presence is taken to indicate that the transplanted marrow's beginning to grow, that a graft seems to be taking place.

Platelets, another name for thrombocytes, break off from megakaryocytes, bone marrow cells that are very, very large—eight to ten times bigger than lymphocytes. Then there are eosinophils, basophils, macrophages. There's plasma, the blood's water. In the bone marrow, there's fat. If any of these components are out of proportion—if there are more of a given type of cell than is normal, or too few—something is probably wrong. Too few platelets mean blood won't clot. Too many immature white cells—blasts—in the peripheral blood indicates leukemia. And as there are two stem cell lines—the myeloid and the lymphoid—so there are two kinds of blasts, myeloblasts and lymphoblasts. You can't always tell them apart, although in order to know which disease is the culprit—myelogenous or lymphatic leukemia, for example—it's necessary to find out, because the type indicates the treatment.

If cells are misshapen, it's an indication of disease: sickle cell anemia, for instance, takes its name from the deformed shape of erythrocytes. If cells are the wrong size, it also means trouble.

Immature cells are bigger, the nucleus gets more condensed, and the cell gets smaller as they mature. Some cell types can't be detected morphologically, by looking at their shape; it's impossible to differentiate between a T and B cell using this method, and therefore the question of whether someone has a T-cell or B-cell lymphoma or leukemia can't be answered by looking through the microscope. Instead, Smith explains, "we make—or get—monoclonal antibodies that will bind to a B cell but not a T cell, or vice versa." And *always* Rappeport's assumption is that the more thoroughly the cause of disease is understood, the better the chance of cure. If not now, later. If not for this patient, then for others to come.

Sometimes, as a result of one of the enormous number of blood diseases, cells look chopped up—"the Waring Blender syndrome," says Rappeport—or get stuck together, or "guillotined." There are cells peculiar to rare diseases that don't exist in a healthy person—severe Gaucher's disease, for example, of which the vast majority of doctors, including hematologists, will never see an actual case.

Into the laboratory lesson Rappeport weaves a lecture, delivered as a chat. It's about the history of hematology and the science of morphology—a methodology that preceded the techniques of molecular biology and exists now alongside them—but he makes identifying the shape of cells sound like an art. "Dr. Moloney," Rappeport says, honoring his senior with the inflection he uses as he says the title, developed important staining techniques, and was brilliant at reading slides, moving the picture around so fast "you'd get seasick." Rappeport claims he thinks other lines of work are worthy, but his reverence for medicine, "our profession," is evident, and he'll speak of and to a doctor he considers incompetent with ruthless disdain.

A couple of yards from where Rappeport sits with his students, Brian Smith stands teasing a fellow, a young woman doing research on cell membranes. "What makes a red cell a red cell?" Smith asks. "That's a philosophical question. Because it expresses hemoglobin?"

"Because it expresses spectrin," she says. Spectrin is a protein red cell membranes—"skeletons"—produce. She goes on at length, talking about glycoproteins and chromosomal regions. It's the language of molecular biology, and everyone at the microscope stops to listen.

In hematology, patient care and basic science are fused. Though the diseases Rappeport addresses and the treatment on which he concentrates are dreadful, the promise of advances is constant. Though their implementation is often halting, they grind along on a foundation of deep and growing knowledge and understanding.

Diana Beardsley has a Ph.D. as well as an M.D.; she is a pediatric hematologist at Yale, and says she can't imagine being anywhere else in these times. The activity and place to which she refers is medicine and science, where, in her tone as much as her telling, everything is possible, or at least everything will be. She talks about the amazing progress against illness that she's seen in her career—less than twenty years so far—and has no patience with doomsaying.

Rappeport says "Diana never gives up." Her specialty is bleeding disorders—hemophilia, mostly—but she sees children with other blood diseases, including leukemia. One fall afternoon, about six, she stopped by to see Rich Frisbee. Rich's mother Christine and his father Rick, and Rappeport, were in Rich's room, where the atmosphere was heavy with concern. It was before the transplant, and Rich had a respiratory infection so severe he was having trouble breathing. He needed oxygen, but the suggestion he receive it frightened his parents, probably because it's so often administered along with a damning prognosis. It scared Rich too. At that point he'd been in the hospital all of the autumn, getting sicker and sicker, thinner and thinner. I visited the hospital each week, and every time I saw him, I was sure he'd die before I could see him again. In the summer he'd been healthy, a tanned, fourteen-year-old boy. Only a couple of months later, I saw him crouched on his bed on his hands and knees, the most nearly comfortable position he could find for his chemotherapy-raw skin and his clogged lungs.

Beardsley, talking in a leisurely way, though she had stopped in on her way home, explained to the Frisbees that the administration of oxygen wasn't a threatening signal, that it was only to make Rich more comfortable. And she told Rich he had control over it. She was very matter-of-fact and very warm. She described the way he'd use it—that it would come through a tube into two prongs he'd insert in his nostrils—"only as far as you'd pick your nose." The Frisbees were reassured, and Rich did recover from the bout that that time, as many other times, looked like it would kill him.

The chemotherapy Rich Frisbee was receiving at this time was *not* part of a bone marrow transplant. It was standard, aggressive treatment for acute leukemia. In Rich's case it couldn't work permanently because the type of leukemia with which he was afflicted affects the stem cell, but the long, expensive hospitalization and the suffering Rich endured were not extraordinary for someone with his disease. The therapy he received was not experimental. Everyone was praying it would work well enough to *allow* a bone marrow transplant. That was his only chance at cure, since the rescue the donor marrow provides means that it's possible to eradicate malignant stem cells. To the Frisbees at this time, the goal was just to reach the point where a bone marrow transplant would be possible. But whether or not the transplant had even been considered, the personal, financial, and social cost would have been the same—or higher—unless Rich had been simply, at the outset, left untreated and allowed to die, without making the effort to extend both hope and life.

After seeing the Frisbees, Beardsley, bespectacled, with pale blond hair pulled back, sat with her overcoat on, talking to Rappeport at the nursing station near Rich's room. She compared notes on how bad his lungs sounded, went over the possibilities and probabilities and the risks of drug treatments, ending with a "Hmm," a sigh and a nod, acknowledgments of difficulty that did not include despair. The discussion had an intellectual component—Beardsley was making sure she hadn't missed anything that would help, and that Rappeport was thinking of everything—but its main function seemed emotional. Beardsley wanted to make sure she was doing all she could for her patient, that every possibility was considered. Later, when it was sure Rich would have a transplant, she continued to talk about options, trying to avoid problems. Walking with Rappeport in the hall or parting from him on the stairs, she'd raise another question. With so much building going on in the hospital, was aspergillus—an airborne fungus released from the excavations of construction projects, and commonly fatal to people with suppressed immune systems—a particular danger? Since Rich's donor was to be one of his sisters, rather than his brother, should the marrow be T-cell-depleted? Would depleting it be taking too much of a risk of leukemic recurrence?

In these conversations Beardsley's manner was calm, but she wasn't a bit detached. This kid's welfare was on her mind and in her heart. To clear need, she was applying complex understanding.

Nearly all the knowledge she can draw on has been, and is, gained incrementally. The parallel to patient care in bone marrow transplants is exact: the possibilities of a particular discovery or an individual attempt at cure, let alone proof of its staying power, aren't known at the time of the original research or hospitalization.

Nevertheless, it's striking how fully absorbed and widely applicable a relatively recent breakthrough can be. When I mentioned Max Perutz's name to Diana Beardsley, she said, "That's where it all began, isn't it?" Perutz won the Nobel Prize for solving the structure of hemoglobin in 1962, the same year Watson and Crick got their award for the discovery of DNA.

Perutz prefaces his most authoritative statements with diffident gestures, but in conversation he gives no hint of self-doubt. He is sure of his knowledge on subjects that range from the safety of the London subway to the structure of hemoglobin. "Oh," he said, his fingers to his forehead, after I told him what I wanted: a précis of his career, and an overview of the whole field. Then he eagerly gave an hour-long disquisition that was completely to the point.

When he began, Perutz says, the idea he would know every atom in hemoglobin was crazy. He'd have dismissed even the thought of it as ridiculous. His work, he says, has been successful "beyond my wildest dreams." He says that what he did, and what he won the Nobel Prize for, was to develop a *method* for solving the structure of proteins. Doing so, he says, was necessary. Without it, we "wouldn't have gained any knowledge of basic biology." Blood's accessibility and malleability led him to hemoglobin; he needed a protein that could be easily obtained and crystallized. Hemoglobin "was just a convenient model for attacking the structure of proteins." X-ray analysis, he says, was "the only possible method of solving the structure of proteins."

The methodology has enormous applicability: For example, says Perutz, "the exciting development of a humanized rat monoclonal antibody against T-cell leukemia, through genetic engineering. And the crucial step in this engineering required a knowledge of the atomic structure of the antibody, which had been obtained by X-ray crystallography." (Smith describes X-ray crystallography as a method of understanding three-dimensional structure.) There's a genetically modified insulin in the works—its modification based on the X-ray detection of the atomic structure of insulin—that would elicit a more rapid response than normal pig or human insulin does. Protein crystallography began, Perutz says, with Bernal and Crowfoot's X-ray diffraction from a crystal of pepsin, an enzyme that breaks down proteins, in 1934. The structure of pepsin, however, Perutz adds, was not solved until quite recently. Now, he goes on, it turns out that the AIDS virus contains a pepsinlike enzyme. "So if you can find a way of inhibiting that enzyme, you would have a promising drug against AIDS. And in fact, several pharmaceutical firms have made such compounds and are testing them now."

Down the hall from Perutz's office, a model of hemoglobin stands on a table in a large room. The place looks like a war room or a planning center for an expedition. A woman works quietly in a corner, there's a chart spread out on a table, and a wide shelf running along the walls holds a variety of models, the double helix being immediately recognizable. The hemoglobin model is larger, at least three feet in diameter. It is a huge, airy mass of detail, of small prongs and branches and globes. The study of it has been Perutz's life's work, and he is sure of the value of his effort. This giant molecule, he explains, clicks backward and forward between two alternative structures every time it takes up oxygen and releases it. (Brian Smith explains the click as "analogous to a light switch. You can turn it on and off, but it's not stable in between.") The mechanism of the switch was the most important result that emerged from his work, Perutz said. There are many other proteins that change their structures in response to chemical stimuli, but until 1988, hemoglobin was the only one in which that change was understood in atomic detail.

"It might seem funny that I've been doing it so long," says Perutz, speaking of his lifelong study, but there was another problem. Several hundred abnormal hemoglobins—mutations—puzzle hematologists. They send samples to Perutz's laboratory, and his group, using X-ray analysis, can explain the clinical abnormalities in atomic terms. If the hemoglobin has too high an oxygen affinity, it leads to too many red cells. If it has a low oxygen affinity, there are too few. Sometimes there's premature destruction.

Then, there's a second, connected line of research. Hemoglobin can act as a receptor for certain drugs, some of which change its oxygen affinity. Through crystallography, Perutz finds out how the receptor works and where the drug goes, allowing chemists to tailor the drug to the protein.

Perutz is a "pure scientist." But he had written, in a review of a book about science, of the value of "tales of pain and sorrow, of love and joy,"[4] and the emotion of the statement, as much as the fame of his accomplishment, made me want to meet him, and to ask him the role of altruism in his work. Most of it, he said, "is curiosity-motivated." He paused, looking down, thinking—Perutz's pauses have the precision and purpose of Beethoven's rests—and then spoke again. "But it would be absolutely marvelous," he said, "if some of my work actually improved the treatment of human disease." Perutz was in his seventies when he talked to me, but his statement had the hope usually associated with the most idealistic youth. At the same time, he has the kind of generous self-assurance that only a long life-time of experience and attainment gives.

Viennese by birth, he is English by lucky accident. Perutz left Austria in the late thirties to continue his education and so was safe when World War II began. His parents and sister got out in time, too; his sister now lives in Vermont. He told me this with sudden gravity, answering my questions about his personal history over lunch he bought for me and ate with me. I sat behind my tray while he, because of his back problems, stood, carving a piece of chicken with dexterity, and with delicacy picked up a stray pea and put it at the edge of his plate. Both his action and his reaction to my inquiries were exact, contained, and appropriate.

Perutz has a manner that would be courtly if it were not also egalitarian. He is careful but not careworn, scrupulous about being factually correct. His attentiveness is so complete it's a challenge. He's alert for new information, listening carefully when I told him what I'd been reading and hearing about gene therapy for severe combined immunodeficiency, an undertaking that, at the time of our meeting, was receiving a great deal of publicity in the United States.

When I asked him if he thought gene therapy was dangerous, he said no. "The children are so ill that even if there's a remote chance of cancer twenty years later, they still would have had twenty years of healthy life." (The cancer he's referring to would, in the case of the experiments we were discussing, be a result of the therapy, as the children's original disease is not malignant.) And actually, he said, he couldn't envision a harmful effect. "It's a cleaner experiment" than a bone marrow transplant, the current accepted therapy for severe combined immunodeficiency, "and less dangerous because it would not lead to graft rejection." And look-ing backward in order to look forward, the "fear of DNA was not justified."[5] Use of techniques involving recombinant DNA are commonplace in biology and medical laboratories now, and until Perutz's statement I had almost forgotten the predictions of disaster that were usual only a decade or so ago.

Max Perutz's laboratory is in Cambridge, a couple of miles from the Cavendish Laboratories, where Watson and Crick discovered DNA—"the secret of life," the tour guide atop an open double-decker bus reverently stated as we rode past the site. On the same ride, she also told us sightseers that the local Catholic church, built at the end of the nineteenth century, was financed by a ballerina whose husband made a fortune by inventing dolls' eyes that opened and shut, that Cambridge would be beneath water in a matter of days were it not for the pumps that cleared the fens, the depth beneath the streets at which Roman roads had been found, and something of the history of the American Cemetery, at which we stopped. It was beautiful there, a perfect example of England's "green and pleasant land," a windy blue sky and smooth grass dotted, at exact intervals, with long lines of white grave markers. I cried for my sister, who hadn't been especially on my mind then until the sight was before me. That day the connectedness of the world seemed both obvious and miraculous.

Perutz is a chemist. At least, that was his original area of expertise. But his Nobel Prize–winning accomplishment involved physics, and has wide biological and medical applicability. His work has something of the developmental quality Rappeport points to in explaining blood cells, and is easier to define than to categorize.

Brian Smith thinks the term "molecular biologist" has been unfairly co-opted by groups of researchers working in basic science, in DNA. "It's a silly term, isn't it? I mean, biochemistry is biology of molecules at the protein level. And molecular biology is sort of the biology of molecules—of nucleic acid molecules. But it's *all* molecules. People interested in DNA grabbed a wonderful term and took it to themselves. And now everyone else who deals with molecules is just a protein chemist or just a biochemist. And not," he whispers, "a molecular biologist." He certainly studies molecules. He also applies learning gleaned from his laboratory and others. Molecular biology, one scientist finally explained to me, after I had been searching for a definition for many months, is "the science based on the belief that all biological function can be explained by the interactions between molecules." It started with Watson and Crick, of course, he said, "but it applies to much more than DNA." I found it interesting that he used the word *belief* in defining his discipline, and revealing. It's true that even the current, rapidly expanding knowledge is a mere window on the unknown, only emphasizing the vastness of it. And what could be "much more than DNA," the tour guide's "secret of life"?

Extrapolation from Watson and Crick's discovery, and Perutz's, is. A sifting of the importance of the flood of data now constantly being published and posited—this is the talent and wisdom for which Smith particularly praises Rappeport. And a broad application of the scientific understanding gained. Although they have never met and have no contact, the line between Perutz and Rappeport is direct and critical, a living example of the history of science and medicine.

When I ask Rappeport for an illustration of the applications of molecular biology in his own work, he says, What of the possibility of heredity in aplastic anemia, for instance? Not only in the very rare known-to-be-genetic types such as Fanconi's anemia, but in more problematic instances? He's talking about his favorite "double hit" theory—or probability—again. This time he's speaking in genetic terms, and the example he uses involves enzymes, ubiquitous molecules. "One of our benzene-induced aplastic anemia patients is a woman who worked at Chrysler, in one of the big plants in the Detroit area. Apparently, after she developed her case, OSHA [Occupational Safety and Health Administration] went in—this was PI (pre-Iacocca) and the plant was a real pit—and made them clean up their act.

"I don't know how many people worked there. One thousand people, two thousand people, five thousand people. Whatever it was. Why is it this one woman develops aplastic anemia? Maybe she got more of the exposure. Maybe she had had some prior hit before, that made her susceptible. But one of the other possibilities is, maybe she was defective in an enzyme that prevented the breakdown of benzene. You'd say, Well, is that all pie in the sky?

"Well, it turns out there is an animal—a rabbit model? I think it's a rabbit model, not a mouse"—Rappeport, relishing his story and apparently telling it casually, is also anguishing over the details—"a model called AH 2, or something like that, defective rabbits—who have an increased susceptibility to benzene toxicity, and are missing a specific enzyme. Never been looked at in humans.

So there's not *proof* there yet. But what are the implications if one finds that kind of thing? Nothing in terms of the treatment of aplastic anemia." But because it could play a role in its prevention, "it raises a major social problem. Which is, if you can now go and test prospective employees for the presence or absence of that enzyme, are you going to deny someone employment who's defective in that enzyme? It's a very interesting, complicated social issue." He nods his head, looking—for him—relaxed. The fact that the predicament's interesting takes the curse off it.

Still, everything about the story, including the answers he suggests and the problems he sees, are, like many aspects of Rappeport's world, the product of the uneasiness that inconclusiveness brings. Often, the knowledge an understanding of molecular biology provides doesn't yet give definitive answers. In his work, there's no more an intellectual resting place than there is an emotional one. A decade and a half after Ricky had been his patient, Rappeport told Sis Stott, "There isn't a day that goes by that Ricky isn't talked about, that his name isn't mentioned." He meant, says Sis, that lessons learned from the treatment of her son led to the saving of other lives, and she is grateful that Ricky is thus remembered. But Rappeport remembers him in other ways that he doesn't articulate.

It wasn't Rappeport, but other people, who first mentioned the Stotts' name to me, and told me a little of their story. Rappeport did not suggest I meet Sis, or encourage me once I had decided to do so. Although he agreed, with a kind of sad force, to my admiring comments about Sis and her family, he volunteered very little about the Stotts. It was just plain hard for him to talk about them. He could not have saved Ricky; the knowledge did not then exist that would have made it possible. And yet, Rappeport feels his loss with regret—with responsibility. It's the paternal in him, a virtue that should be remembered, I think, despite the opprobrium the suffix "istic" brings to the meaning of the word. It is, after all, a good thing to be a loving parent, a condition that often involves a wish for omnipotence and a feeling of guilt when we are helpless. When my mother, in the worst of her grief, said, "I guess I couldn't have kept Roberta from getting leukemia," she wasn't being entirely sardonic. She was mourning, going over and over the steps that led to the incomprehensible and unacceptable. She had not been able to protect her child, and she was punishing herself for that.

Peter Benelli is headmaster of Thayer Academy, Rappeport's alma mater. He was not at the school when Rappeport was, but they are friends. Thayer gave Rappeport an Alumni Achievement Award, and at the reception Rappeport made a remark to the headmaster that stuck with Benelli. Benelli repeated it to me with imitative force. "I never forget a patient who died," Rappeport had volunteered into an evening of pleasantries, tensing himself and raising his voice. "Never."

FOUR

Discovery

*R*appeport was a primary participant in the first full correction of Wiskott-Aldrich syndrome,[1] an effort that resulted in a better understanding of the stem cell's function. In this instance, analysis of a patient's treatment and his continuing illness pointed to new theoretical understanding and then—with the same little boy—to cure. "It wasn't a planned attack," Rappeport says. "It was looking carefully at what happened, coming to a conclusion, and trying to solve the problem."

The problem, in 1976, was trying to cure Patrick Hough, then three and a half. His older brother Christopher had died of Wiskott-Aldrich syndrome, a disease that, because it is on the X chromosome, is passed, like hemophilia (or, for that matter, color blindness), from mother to son and that, without a bone marrow transplant, invariably kills its victims in childhood—nearly always before the age of ten.

Children with Wiskott-Aldrich syndrome have insufficient and abnormal platelets and T cells, and are therefore subject to constant and extreme bleeding and infection. Because only boys are afflicted, Beverly, second in the family, was never in danger. Scott, the oldest, was also spared. Pamela Hough, their mother, was pregnant with Patrick when Christopher was diagnosed. The doctors didn't know what was wrong at first, and when they did they didn't explain it clearly to the Houghs. Christopher was bleeding internally, his eyes were crossing, and he had terrible eczema.

"He was very ill," Pam says, but that was all that was clear to her. During the first hospitalization, Pam would catch a doctor in the hall at eight o'clock at night, "and it'd be 'Oh, yes, I've been meaning to speak to you.' And you'd stand there, and they'd mumble all this encyclopedia at you. It took me a long time to realize what was going on, and the prognosis," she says. "Those things don't occur in everyday common life. One of your children is stricken with it, and it's overwhelming. It was totally overwhelming."

Patrick was diagnosed in infancy. He was premature, not because he had Wiskott-Aldrich but perhaps, Pam thinks, because Christopher did. She was worn out during her pregnancy with Patrick, running back and forth between one desperately sick child in the hospital and his young sister and brother at home. "I just didn't have the time to take care of myself like I should have."

Patrick almost died of pneumonia when he was only a few weeks old. Because children with Wiskott-Aldrich syndrome have abnormal lymphocytes, their bodies can't fight infections effectively, but Patrick survived this episode and the ones that followed. And so, for several years, Pam Hough had two acutely ill children to take care of and to feel for. Eczema tormented them. Patrick, she says, "would open his mouth and his skin would split and bleed. And there were big clumps on his head. I used to put out two bathtubs, and give them oatmeal baths. And then rub them down with tar cream. And then put little nightcaps on them and cover their hands up, because they would scratch so hard they would bleed. And the skin would get infected and have kind of a smell, an odor to it. It was really hard. And his eyes used to—it was awful. I remember one time I went to Children's Hospital and they had to clean all the stuff away from his eyes; I didn't want to rip away his skin or anything wiping at his eyes, so crusty from the eczema."

Rappeport was never Christopher's doctor; he first met the Houghs only a few months before Patrick's transplant. In the meantime, for both little boys, there was hospitalization after hospitalization. Christopher was in the hospital for *months* with chicken pox. In the hospital, there was "testing. There were tests. You know, research. And they would give them other tests, and give them shots other times. I don't know why. Poor Chrissie." Later, "he'd go into the hospital, and they'd have an incision in his neck for the IV; his veins had collapsed. And it was just too painful. So I said, 'No, I don't want it. That's it.' " She took him home, and eventually he died. There was never any hope for him, because the only possible cure was a bone marrow transplant, and Christopher did not have a compatible donor.

Patrick did—his sister Beverly. She was six and seven years old when Christopher was dying, and remembers it well. "I don't remember when he got Wiskott-Aldrich. I just know he always had it. I remember celebrating his birthdays in the hospital. We'd all get dressed up and bring his cake and everything and have his cake in the hospital. It was just an awful time. I remember my parents weren't around. We stayed at the O'Briens' house; they live two houses down." She talks about the O'Brien children, still close friends, and about Mrs. O'Brien. "She was just wonderful. And God, I remember the way Christopher always looked. His face was all broken out, and his eyes and his mouth. And he had skinny, skinny legs and arms. And a big belly. He was always sick. He and Paddy were always sick. It's just awful, how Scott and I are healthy, and they are sick. And I think that's kind of what's the most disturbing about it. It just didn't seem right. They were so little. We were little, too. But it just never seemed right; it was odd."

When Beverly was a donor, she had a guardian ad litem; Massachusetts then required a court hearing to ensure that a minor donor was not being coerced. "I remember my mom saying, 'You don't have to do this, you don't have to do this.' " Beverly was a little girl, barely school age, but she had seen Christopher die, and she knew what she wanted, though her mother told her that her life was in danger.

The risk to the donor of any serious injury is extremely remote, but it exists. Infection is a possibility, and although Rappeport has never heard of an anesthesia-related death befalling a bone marrow donor, it could happen. He told me this during our first meeting, when he examined me. In this conversation he also offered to lie for me, if I didn't want to serve. If that was the case, he said, he'd preserve peace in my family by telling them, for example, that the match was not good enough after all. He says this to all adult donors, in order to prevent undue family pressure or an irremediable rift.

Reality is pressure enough, however. When Beverly Hough was eight years old, she knew enough to be appalled by the idea that she had any choice. "I'm like, 'What?'" She contorts her face, expressing her incredulity at her mother's scrupulousness. "What do you mean, I don't have to do this? Patrick's going to die. You don't say you don't have to do it." A psychologist examined her, and found her intelligence high, her understanding good, her altruism well developed.

In court, "I felt really scared. Joel was there, and my parents and my lawyer. It was really strange. I had my lawyer, and I was so young. I remember the judge took me into his room and gave me candy as he was talking to me, and he was really nice."

Beverly told me this years after the fact, on an evening in late December, a Christmas tree in the corner of the room where we sat. "I was looking for Christmas things the other day, like tape and name tags, and I found the court papers. God! They wrote down everything you say! I'd never seen those before. I remember going to court, though. I remember getting so scared when I had to go up on the witness stand. But it was fine, they just said, Do you understand? and I pretty much did."

Patrick Hough underwent two bone marrow transplants. The first took place on May 25, 1976, and didn't work. At first it seemed to. "His counts were rising," Rappeport says. "His white count and retic." This is short for reticulocytes, young red cells. Then Patrick developed an infection, and "in late June, his crit dropped." *Crit* is short for *hematocrit*, the measure of the volume of packed red cells ("just a percentage of how much of a tube of blood is red," Rappeport says), and is part of the lingo in which hematological patients become fluent. Bactrim, the antibiotic with which Patrick was being treated, can cause a drop in the hematocrit, so Rappeport discontinued it, but the drug wasn't the source of the problem. Patrick continued to need platelets. The ones his body produced were not from Beverly's marrow. They were the small, dysfunctional ones characteristic of Wiskott-Aldrich syndrome, and didn't survive well. There were other ways to tell the graft hadn't taken. The red blood cells were type O, Patrick's original blood type, rather than A, Beverly's. (Unlike people who undergo solid organ transplants, people who have bone marrow transplants do not have to have the same blood type as their donor. In a successful bone marrow transplant, the new bone marrow, from the donor, determines the blood type.) In addition, chromosomal analysis showed a high percentage of the granulocytes to be male.

By nine months after the transplant, there was no evidence of any donor cells. Nevertheless, Patrick's eczema had cleared. It was the preparatory immunosuppressants that did it, Rappeport says. "And that's still interesting. No one knows what eczema is, or why it went away in Patrick's case." Eczema is presumed to be an antoimmune disease. "In autoimmunity," says Brian Smith, "the body makes a normal immune reaction—but inappropriately, to oneself." It's thought-provoking that suppressing the immune system cured eczema.

It's possible that a variety of autoimmune diseases—a large classification, afflicting huge numbers of people—might be amenable to bone marrow transplantation. Aplastic anemia, for example, has an autoimmune component in some cases. Rappeport has a patient, a druggist living in New York, whose graft failed but whose marrow returned, apparently as a result of the immunosuppressive preparatory regimen. Rappeport and Smith both say that bone marrow transplantation "is an immunological procedure, not an oncological one."

Patrick, however, had not been cured. Other than clearing up his eczema, the obvious positive accomplishments of the first transplant were few. The nurses weaned him from the bottle and taught him to use the potty. "Well, boys," said Fred Rosen, a senior immunologist, to Rappeport and his colleagues, "you've just accomplished a $250,000 toilet training." The remark, says Rappeport, was intended to break the tension, then running very high. Patrick was going to die. He was given platelet transfusions periodically—Pam remembers it as every day, and recalls, also, that both her little boys were always covered with bruises—while the doctors decided what to do. "We evaluated him extensively," Rappeport says. "His red cells were his own. Myeloid cells his own. B cells were his own."

And then, there was the clue. "T cells—which he had not had before—were donor, but over a period of months they began to fall in number. And with that observation we realized he had engrafted only what wasn't there, and that not permanently. Everything else came back."

It certainly hadn't been obvious that this would happen. In

Wiskott-Aldrich syndrome the problem seems to be more a deficiency than a defect. Illness comes from an insufficiency of working
cells rather than from the aggressiveness of malignant ones. It
would seem, therefore, that a transplant should be done as it would
be for a patient with aplastic anemia, rather than as it would be for
someone with leukemia—the treatment would be one of replacement rather than eradication.

Nevertheless, the fact that two cells—absent T cells and defective platelets—caused Wiskott-Aldrich pointed to the need to
eliminate the abnormal pluripotent stem cell. Since T cells descend
from the lymphoid stem cell and platelets from the myeloid stem
cell, it was necessary to go all the way back to the root of blood
production. To create "space, not physical space, but some other
kind of hematopoietic space," Rappeport explains. He reasoned
that it was the preparation that had been faulty in Patrick's first
transplant. Then, he had used only immunosuppressive drugs—
cyclophosphamide, a customary part of the preparatory regimen,
and, "We threw in cytosine arabinoside (ARA-C) because we
thought we'd get more immunosuppression with it." ARA-C is a
commonly used chemotherapeutic agent, unpleasantly familiar to
cancer patients.

Rappeport pressed for a second transplant, to be done this
time with more intensive preparation, especially with total body
irradiation, so as to eradicate the stem cell. (Nowadays in patients
with Wiskott-Aldrich, the drug busulfan is usually used instead of
radiation.) Because laboratory tests showed that the first transplant
had sensitized Patrick to Beverly's marrow, graft rejection was
likely. The protocol for the second transplant therefore included
procarbazine, another chemotherapeutic drug that suppresses bone
marrow function (including immunity), and antihuman lymphocyte serum, an antiserum produced in rabbits that, given intravenously, binds to lymphocytes—mostly T cells—thus suppressing
the immune system. Rappeport's colleagues, especially his superiors, were reluctant, at the very least, to go along with a second
attempt. "They thought Patrick wouldn't survive it," says Rappeport, "and called us Nazis."

"Patrick was a very important case in the history of medicine,"
Fred Rosen says, "because it was the first time a genetic defect was
cured by bone marrow transplantation—where you were replacing
something that was bad with something that was normal. That
statement would be incorrect without that last bit, because before

that, severe combined immunodeficiency had been corrected by bone marrow transplantation. So Patrick was a *very* important case in showing that you could wipe out the abnormal and replace it with normal cells. That had never been done before. And I remember doing that, we were frightened to death . . . because we were removing everything. We just—destroyed him. You know, destroyed his bone marrow—the bad bone marrow."[2]

But after the first transplant, Patrick's body wasn't able to utilize transfused platelets. Even those gathered from a single donor didn't work; this is a highly specialized blood-banking resource Rappeport frequently has to resort to for his patients, who, through multiple transfusions, often build up antibodies to the very cells they need. In addition, Patrick wasn't eating well and had fevers, both symptoms of immunodeficiency. It was clear that he would die without a second transplant. Parkman and Rappeport said so, and their superiors and the Houghs agreed to their proposal.

Time has proved them right. "This treatment of the Wiskott-Aldrich syndrome may be a model for the correction of other genetically determined immune and hematologic bone-marrow disorders," says the *New England Journal of Medicine* article[3] in which they reported the case, and this has turned out to be largely true. Patrick Hough's experience is a success story, but one with high emotional and physical costs for him and his family.

Pam Hough is an exceptionally pretty woman, with soft blond hair, high cheekbones, and green eyes, but she isn't looking for glamour. All she wants is normalcy, although she also says, "Anything's a disorder today. Curly hair's a disorder." Of the fright and sadness and the effort to save Patrick, with the long, long hospitalizations, when the grief over Christopher was still fresh, she says, "It was a long time ago. I'm trying to think what our reaction was." She has talked about how terrible it was, and how pathetic. How she would stay at the hospital each day until Patrick took his bowel prep, the disgusting-tasting gastrointestinal antibiotic. "And oh, 'My tummy! My tummy!' You know, you're nauseous, and you know you're not going to hold it—and he'd throw it up. And they would make him do it three times, and after the third time they wouldn't make him do it again. But we'd try to help him get through his bowel prep. Then we'd leave for the night. He had a color TV and a telephone, all his sterilized toys and food."

There were nurses who didn't look after him properly, who let him lie in his own vomit and diarrhea, so that Pam, coming in to see him, would scrub and dress in the requisite way—it took her ten minutes—and then go in and clean her child, flinging the filthy sheets out of the room. Most of the nurses were good during the second transplant, she says, and there were some good ones the first time. "But there were a couple that just— I can remember Patrick's father going in and having a fight with one of them. I can remember calling one of the doctors and saying, 'I think you better get over there. Kevin just went flying out of the house.' " (Kevin and Pam Hough are divorced now.)

Beverly says that there were nurses who, during Patrick's first transplant, "wouldn't change his sheets. It was awful. And it drove my parents crazy, because what could they do? Except for complain, and then the nurses get spiteful toward you. There were some really good nurses, too. I remember Joleen and Barbara. They were really nice. But the other ones just didn't really care, for some reason."

Pam Hough treasures her privacy—talking to me was an act of great generosity. "What I wanted," she said, speaking of the time of the finally successful transplant, of a life that had for years revolved around catastrophic illness and the hospital, "was just to come home and mow the lawn, cook a meal, and just get back with the family. More than anything. Just to have Patrick back home." "Paddy," she calls him at other times. And "Pat." "There was so much time consumed with Chris," she says. "Paddy was just kind of left on the kitchen table with his blanket, and we'd do whatever we had to do with Christopher."

Pam says, "I realize now, talking to my daughter—she says, 'You know, you're not the only one who went through it.' " Beverly has not yet been tested to see if she is a carrier, but it is now possible for her to find out. "We can diagnose carriers," says Fred Rosen, "with confidence." That is, with reasonable reliability but not certainty. Should Beverly turn out to be a carrier, there is also a prenatal test for the disease, making abortion an option. "We can tell for sure by twenty weeks of gestation," Fred Rosen says.[4]

Beverly is a beautiful young woman, fair and wide-eyed, but she has no apparent vanity. The emotion she most expresses is protectiveness. She says that she would not have a child if there were even the slightest chance that he could have Wiskott-Aldrich syndrome. "I just couldn't go through that again," Beverly says. She says of her mother, simply and with assurance, "She's a good person. She was a wreck, physically and mentally, because Christopher died, and Paddy was going through the same thing. But she wouldn't show that to us. I think my mother's very strong. If I were her, I think I would have fallen apart. I couldn't have done that and still lived."

Beverly saved Patrick, and she is full of concern for him now, alert to any slights he receives. "His legs are really scarred and everything from the shunts. And I know when he was younger the kids used to give him a hard time about that. I think that was probably the most painful experience that he can remember." There was the time, for example, that she drove him to the local mall. Patrick ran in to do a quick errand, and Beverly waited in the car. "And he walked by, and he walks with a limp, and I remember girls laughing and imitating him. I think that's the most painful kind of experience, when people don't understand." She is anxious about the possibility of any more bad health befalling him. The limp is the result of a clot that formed around the shunt he had during the transplant. The clot extended into the arteries, Rappeport says, preventing one leg from growing properly for a while. "He then developed collaterals—arteries around the obstruction—and then there was arterial flow; both legs grew." But one leg is still shorter than the other.

Both Hickman lines and Thomas shunts are means of vascular access, but Hickman lines are inserted in the main vein in the chest, whereas Thomas shunts are inserted in an artery and vein in the upper thigh and groin and form a loop outside the skin. Rappeport refers to the safer and more efficient Hickman lines as "a great advance." Patrick's bad experience with a shunt proves his point.

In addition to the leg problem the clot caused, Patrick developed a tumor in his leg that looked malignant but turned out to be benign. This happened years after the transplant—when Patrick was in sixth grade—and was a terrible scare. People with Wiskott-Aldrich syndrome sometimes die of tumors, as well as from bleeding and infection, and people who have had bone marrow transplants sometimes develop tumors as a result of the profound immunosuppression chemotherapy and radiation cause. Moreover, surgery to remove the tumor caused excruciating pain. Patrick wouldn't let visitors touch the bed he was in, let alone touch him. He has also had cataracts. And despite his normal, perhaps high, intelligence, he has trouble reading and writing because of learning disabilities, presumably caused by the battering his body took so he could live. But when Pam Hough told Rappeport she was worried about the amount of radiation Patrick had received, he told her to go to the library and take out some books on Hiroshima.

As the years have gone by, there have been Patrick's cataracts, a problem Pam categorizes as "relatively minor," and the operations on his legs, which she describes as ordeals, and always her ongoing worry—the whole family's worry—about possible repercussions from the enormous, intense dose of radiation. She speaks highly of Rappeport, says he was always available to answer a question, always told her to bring Patrick right in when there was a problem, but without saying anything bad about anybody Pam Hough tells about the aggravation that comes with endless dealings with doctors. She tells of taking her child for a doctor's appointment, one in which he was to be measured for a growth study. She got so tired of waiting that she just couldn't stand it anymore and, with Patrick, went home.

"They were all very good," she says of the doctors, but right through her telling Pam indicates, sometimes just with a hand gesture, a seconds-long imitation of dismissal or brusqueness or lack of feeling she endured under the more or less constantly horrendous conditions of drawn-out critical, but potentially curable, illness. "It was awful," Pam says, and Beverly, talking separately, says, too, "I can't explain it. It was awful." And that seems just the right explanatory, clarifying word. What happened to the Houghs was hard, and sad, and painful.

Patrick is healthy now, but he is short, also presumably as a result of the radiation he received. Patrick is about five feet, two inches, though his mother and father are both tall and Beverly is six feet. Scott is a huge guy, six foot six, a professional football player. Patrick, too, likes sports. He shoots baskets, plays floor hockey, wrestles. He thinks he would like to be a gym teacher, perhaps for special-needs kids. It's work he likes; he baby-sits for two retarded people, twins.

Patrick is quiet and gentle. But, says Beverly, "he has a lot to say." To her. "We go out shopping, because he likes me to pick out clothes for him, and he picks out clothes for me. And we just go out and drive around. He likes that. He likes to talk and has a lot of feelings and a lot of emotions, but he never just lets himself go and say it. He'll talk to me, because we have this weird connection." She doesn't know if it has anything to do with her having been his donor, but she says, "We're really, really close. I could sit and talk with Patrick for hours and hours and hours, and we won't get bored. With Scott you can talk about football, but with Paddy you can talk about anything."

Scott and Beverly both think Patrick is very strong. They comment on his intelligence and his resiliency. Beverly says, "He's smart. He can do anything. And whatever he does, he'll do well. Because he wants it so bad. I don't know if it has all come from his past experiences or whatever. But he's very, very determined—and what he wants to do, he'll do. He doesn't get discouraged."

Rappeport's unwillingness to allow himself to become discouraged allowed for increased knowledge and saved Patrick Hough. An associate who no longer works directly with Rappeport says, "You loved working with Joel because you knew he'd keep the patient alive." This is said without the slightest irony; it's a simple statement of fact. This doctor doesn't want to spend his whole life in the hospital. He likes getting out and doing other things, and when he worked with Rappeport, he could do so with a free mind. He did much of the laboratory work when he and Rappeport were together, but he says, "What Joel did with Wiskott-Aldrich is every bit as much science as cloning a gene."

Rappeport says the Wiskott-Aldrich experience was like gene transfer, in a way. "You're taking an exogenous source of the gene— cloned by mother nature, rather than in the laboratory—but you *are* putting in a new gene."

Frank Grosveld is a Dutchman who now lives in England. He went there over a decade ago to pursue his scientific work, and he is now world-famous for his ongoing part in the progress of gene transfer. His specialty is gene expression: finding a way to see to it that a gene, once inserted in a body, does what it's supposed to do, in the way it's intended to do it. These genes are not "cloned by mother nature" as Rappeport puts it.

Grosveld's work is experimental, and he works with mice, but the goal, of course, is the cure of disease in human beings. Instead of using a donor's healthy marrow, the patient's own faulty cellular material would be altered in the laboratory and then reinserted, resulting in the eradication of disease. Rappeport says that introducing the properly functioning gene through a conventional transplant is "practically the same thing" as the just-beginning-to-happen gene transfer, and his statement makes the connection and continuum clear. There are obvious differences, however. Although the complicated new technology is incomplete and unproven, implementing it is "a cleaner experiment," as Max Perutz says, because using the patient's own marrow eliminates the possibility of GVH. And the problem of finding a donor—particularly acute in genetic disease, where many family members are likely to have the same problem—doesn't exist, since the patient would use his or her own marrow.

Nevertheless, Grosveld and the other scientist with whom he's most closely associated—Richard Mulligan in the United States, the MacArthur fellow whose work consists primarily of figuring out how to get the genes into the cells—have a reputation for wholesome caution, for integrity. They don't want to rush into a human experiment that could do more harm than good, or even into one that might do nothing and thus teach nothing. Still, Grosveld's work puts him so far on the cutting edge that I expected his personality to match the metaphor.

He walked into our meeting wearing khaki pants, an open-necked purple shirt, and Reeboks. In early middle age, he is handsome. He is tall, bearded, and fair, with blue eyes that, in shape and color, indicate his country of origin. His natural gaze is the unblinking stare. Like virtually everyone I have chosen to write about in this book, he is intense. Before we got started on the subject of our discussion—the promise of gene transfer—he said he wanted to make sure I would present the facts about preventing the diseases that the fruits of his research may cure. Was I aware of prenatal testing and the option of abortion? Because genetic disease can be terrible, and the ones we were talking about, he said, certainly caused dreadful suffering, best avoided.[5]

That cannot always be, however. Often, in genetic disease, there is no family history to serve as a warning. Wiskott-Aldrich syndrome is an extremely rare disease—there are only a handful of cases every year in the world—but genetic disease will always be with us, a fact guaranteed by the process of mutation, which is an essential factor in evolution and thus ensures the perpetuation of the species.

More and more, however, the causes of hereditary illnesses are losing their mystery, and the cure of people stricken with them is increasing. The methodology for this seemingly magical change is concrete but not formulaic. Rappeport believes his success with Wiskott-Aldrich syndrome is representative of a kind of experience that is virtuous, endangered, and necessary: clinical research—learning through the attempt to cure.

*   *   *

Nancy Cahillane, like Pam Hough, had never heard of Wiskott-Aldrich syndrome until Brian Murphy, her child, was stricken with it. But in 1983, seven years after Rappeport and his colleagues had figured out how to save Patrick Hough, he knew what to do for Brian Murphy. He had by then transplanted five other children with Wiskott-Aldrich syndrome, only one of whom—a boy whose donor was a genetic half-match—died. Bone marrow transplants were now proven therapy for Wiskott-Aldrich syndrome, if the patient had a donor.

Nancy had just finished high school when she found she was pregnant. Bill Murphy, her boyfriend, was away at college, and she says she thought it would be better not to get married then, to wait until he'd graduated. But long before Bill finished school Nancy learned about Brian's disease, and very soon she was spending all her time taking her baby to the hospital and staying with him there. And once that was her life, "I just didn't feel the same about Billy. It was weird. All my interest just went to Brian. And that was what we dealt with, and that was just the way it was."

Brian had eczema right from the start; at his six-week checkup the pediatrician gave Nancy a cream to smooth on the rash. When she brought the baby back a week later, "he had all these little dots all over him. I had no clue what it was." They were petechiae, evidence of bleeding under the skin. "Dr. Franklin took a little bit of blood in the office, and I went home, and about an hour and a half later he called me and said, 'Take him right in to Children's Hospital.' " Nancy lives in a Boston suburb, half an hour from its famous hospitals. "I went with my sister and her husband. And we're sitting there, and they took him, and a while later they came back. And all they said to me was, 'Well, it's not leukemia.' And then, I just lost it. I mean, I had no clue that they were even thinking anything near leukemia." It was six months before Brian was diagnosed, and by then Nancy had settled into a routine. The petechiae, she says, were a blessing, because they served as a warning that Brian needed a transfusion. "We'd go in in the morning around nine, and you couldn't preorder platelets, because they couldn't give them to him unless the count was below a certain amount, but it always was. They'd give him a finger stick, and then hours and hours later they'd shoot the platelets in him, and then they'd take another finger stick to make sure the count had gone up, and then we'd go home."

Nancy interrupts her story to explain how platelets are collected from donors: "What you do is, you sit down and you're connected to one arm and the other arm." That is, both arms are connected to a pheresis machine. "They take out your blood, they spin out the platelets, and they give you your blood back. So you can give platelets like once a week. You don't have to wait long like you do when you give regular blood." Actually, a donor can give platelets more than once a week, because pheresis, the process Nancy describes, returns the blood's more slowly regenerating components while taking out only that which will quickly return. But it's an arduous procedure, in which the donor must sit still for hours, with both arms restrained. Platelet donors are heroes to blood bank personnel and patients alike, and many people do it, coming in week after week out of pure altruism.

After a while, the platelets weren't enough to keep Brian going. He became resistant to them. Most people who receive multiple blood transfusions ultimately build up antibodies to the very cells they need, so that sooner or later the therapy stops working. And children with Wiskott-Aldrich syndrome are unable to utilize platelets properly. At first, Brian got platelets once a week, "then it was twice a week, then it was three times a week he was getting the platelets, and it just wasn't cuttin' it. They just weren't staying up. Something was eating them," Nancy says. "He needed them every day."

The next step, when Brian was eleven months old, was removal of his spleen. Rappeport was not yet involved, but he explains the spleen's functions as "multiple. Most consistently, it has a filtering function. It also has some immunological function and some hematological function. As part of normal development, bone marrow does grow there—not in adults but in fetuses and newborns." There's a lot of debate, he says, about when to take it out, but "normal people who've lost spleens in automobile accidents function pretty normally," and so it seems reasonable to remove it "if it's hyperfunctional and destroying too much." This was the reason for surgery in Brian's case, the emblem of which he displays with proud gravity, lifting his T-shirt in order to point out the scar running halfway around his midriff. "The way they explained it to me," Nancy says, "is that spleens are like little filters. The blood gets filtered through the screen, so if something in the spleen was eating away at the platelets, taking it out would let them run smoothly."

"The spleen's interesting," says Brian Smith. "It's sort of two things. There's white pulp and red pulp in the spleen. The red pulp is where the red blood cells go through. That's where they get molded, and membrane comes off their surface, and all that good stuff to keep your red cells neat and clean. The white pulp is basically lymph node. A giant lymph node. In fact, one problem with having your spleen taken out when you're a small child, either because you're in a car accident or because someone's in there taking your appendix out and nicks your spleen and so has to remove it at the same time, or you have a disease that wipes out your spleen, like sickle cell anemia," is that you lose a necessary defense against infection. The reason sickle cell anemia destroys the spleen is that the red cells are misshapen—sickle-shaped, instead of round—and as they go through the spleen they "get stuck," Smith says, destroying the spleen by the time a patient is one or two years old. And if you don't have a spleen when you're a child, "You can die very rapidly from overwhelming bacterial infections. And that's because the spleen is not just *a* lymph node but it's a lymph node that is very specialized for doing a variety of things that seem to be very important when you are, say, two to ten years old. Probably it's less important by the time you're twenty years old. It does a lot of your initial antibody production against sugars, against carbohydrates.

"It turns out that in a lot of the old-fashioned standard pneumonias," those that existed "before we started playing around with people, the little bacteria have a sugar coat around the outside. And what you do is you make antibodies to that, to the carbohydrate coat on the outside of the bacteria, and that's what clues the rest of your immune system to eat the bacteria and get rid of them. And the place where you predominantly make those antibodies is the spleen." Therefore, people who haven't made the antibodies—people with sickle cell anemia, for example, or children like Brian Murphy who lose their spleens when they're very young—need to take an antibiotic, probably for the rest of their lives.

The splenectomy seemed to work for a while, Nancy says. "After they took out his spleen they kept testing him, and the platelets were great, and this went on for seven or eight months, so I was like psyched. I'm like, This is it, it's over, it was the spleen." But then the counts started to plummet. "It wasn't the spleen, obviously. So then, back to the old drawing board, he was going back to the clinic again. I was there every day. From nine o'clock, and we used to get home at five-thirty in the afternoon. We'd sit, and I'd walk him, and I mingled with people, and this one had this, and 'Oh, your son's sick.' In fact," says Nancy, her youth and resiliency in evidence throughout the telling, "there was a Patrick Brian in there, where he was a Brian Patrick." Nancy was nineteen, her experience limited to family life—one of no particular privilege—in a small town. "You know," she says, without any regard for her unusual position, "we all had one thing in common— our kids were sick."

The only thing to be done for Brian now was a bone marrow transplant. But when it was mentioned to Nancy, she cried. "I knew that usually they use a sibling." Her months and months in the hospital had been an education. "So I said, 'Well, I'm going to have another baby.' But the doctor said, 'Nancy, you can't guarantee that even if you had another one, you'd have it in time, and it would even match Brian.' I'm like, *'Fine.'* " In fact, and despite some ethicists' doubts, families do, of course, conceive babies in the hope that the child will be able to serve as a donor. Sometimes they're successful: One of Rappeport's Wiskott-Aldrich patients received his healthy marrow from such a sibling. When Nancy recalls her proposal, and the doctor's response, her tone is sarcastic and despairing, but the rendition is mitigated by the happy outcome and by the time that has passed. "It's so hard to remember. I'm glad it's hard to remember."

There is a 5 percent chance of a parent matching a child exactly at the HLA locus. Still, the call came. "They said, 'Bill matched him *exact.*' The doctors were flippin' out, because I don't think they'd ever seen, in Children's, a parent match like that." Fred Rosen says he has never heard of another instance. "The father and mother shared a haplotype." (A haplotype is a group of alleles; alleles are alternative forms of a gene.) "Brian got the unshared haplotype from the father, the shared haplotype from the mother, so he matched his father perfectly. . . . That's very unusual. That's a 1-in-5,000 chance, for that to happen. That was just lucky. I haven't seen that again. Or before."[6]

"They explained it to me in colors," Nancy says. "I guess I was like blue and green, and I passed on my green to Brian. And Billy was red and green, and he passed on his red. So Billy and Brian were both red and green. I went in the next day and I said, 'Maureen'—this was his primary nurse, I can't remember her last name, she'll kill me—'he's an exact—' And she said, 'Nancy, there must be some mistake. A parent doesn't match.' So she sat me down and came back in. 'I'm sorry, you're right.' Everyone was like, psyched."

Including Billy. "I was at school at the time. At Mass Maritime." On Cape Cod. "And you had to stay there all the time, because it's like a military school. I knew he was really sick [Bill is speaking of the time before the transplant] but we didn't really know what it was for a long time. It was hard to concentrate on anything. My schoolwork suffered. Whenever I would get a chance—on the weekends—I always went in to see him." He was on a mandatory summer training cruise when the word came that he matched Brian. When I asked Bill Murphy if the fact that he and Nancy hadn't been married, and weren't living together, might have influenced him against serving as a donor, he was not so much offended as flabbergasted. "The fact that me and Nancy weren't together wasn't even a consideration. Just the fact that I could help Brian, because he was so sick. That was the only thing on my mind."

Brian spends every weekend with his father. "If Billy had run out on me," Nancy says, "Brian wouldn't be alive."

Bill Murphy, one of seven children, lives with his parents and those of his brothers and sisters who aren't yet married in a small house down the street from Nancy and Brian's apartment. A big picture of Brian sits on a living room table. "We're very proud of him," his grandfather says. Bill's sister Sheila, a nurse, standing in the kitchen where Bill and I sit, says, "I remember I went to get Billy when Brian was sick." She reaches into a cabinet for the dish in which she's about to microwave her dinner. "I remember when he got sick." Then she puts her food down, and speaks with great firmness. "I never thought he would die, though."

"I don't remember if they ever said that he would die," Bill says. "We knew that it was very serious, that there was a possibility. But I always kind of blocked it out, I think. Like Sheila. We didn't let ourselves believe it, I guess."

Everyone in his family "was very supportive" and went to visit Brian, as Bill did—although, he says, "That's the most depressing place I've ever been, is that hospital. All those poor little kids. And so many of them didn't make it. It was just so sad up there. I tried not to get to know anybody. I couldn't take it. It was enough to deal with what I was dealing with."

I too hated the hospital. Everywhere I looked, there were

people who were dying or in danger of it. Brian Smith once asked me why I hated the hospital, but as soon as I began to reply, he understood. I said hospitals had the feeling of an earlier time. Ironically, cost considerations that are partly the result of improved lifesaving technology mandate that nowadays only very seriously ill people are hospital patients—in tertiary-care facilities, at least—for long.

Nevertheless Nancy, Bill Murphy says, made friends with people, with the nurses and doctors and the other parents.

In the first months of Brian's life, Nancy had not met Rappeport, but "I'd seen and heard of him from other people in the hospital. Which was *very* high. I mean, everyone talked about 'Dr. Rappeport.' " Her tone implies awe.

Years after the transplant, her faith in Rappeport is intact, and when she's worried about two lumps she's discovered—one in Brian's back, and another on his knee—she brings him to the Yale clinic.

At nine, Brian is stocky, blond, and tanned. He has round cheeks and a pointed chin. He is wearing shorts, as are his grandmother, Pearl Cahillane, and his mother, Nancy Cahillane. He has on a Teenage Mutant Ninja Turtles wristwatch. Nancy says she has one, too. Rappeport describes Nancy as "very attractive." Nancy, still in her twenties, is short, slim, and shapely. She wears big, blue-framed glasses, two necklaces, several rings, and heart-shaped, dangling pink earrings that match her sleeveless shirt. Her pants are white, accentuating her tan, and her hair is streaked blond.

"You got thin," she says to Rappeport. "I got thin, did you notice?" A few minutes earlier she'd greeted him with a hug.

"I don't think he expected me to hug him," Nancy says to Pearl, when Rappeport steps out of the room. "He held his hand out like he expected to shake hands." When her mother questions the practicality of traveling from Boston to New Haven for a checkup, Nancy says, "I'll go anywhere he tells me. If he tells me to go to *Chicago*, I'll go there."

She gives Rappeport a picture of Brian. It is from the local Little League and is in the form of a baseball card. The back lists Brian's statistics: He is no. 13, is 4 feet 2 inches tall, and weighs 65 pounds. His team is the Blue Jays, and he plays shortstop. He throws right.

Brian's favorite sport, however, is football, and his mother has made a point of bringing him to Rappeport before the season begins. Brian is to play, as usual, in the Pop Warner League, and Nancy wants to make sure the lumps she's discovered aren't anything to worry about. Rappeport feels them and doesn't make much of it. The one on Brian's knee feels like bone, he says. Reminds him of a party game, he says. Remember it? You turn off all the lights and feel each other's legs, trying to figure out if you're touching a girl or a boy. The boys all had bumps on their shins.

"I never heard of that game," Nancy says, holding out her leg.

"It was a fifties game," says Rappeport, and steps into the hall to bring in another doctor, the chief of pediatric surgery.

Dr. John Seashore, accompanied by a house officer and a medical student, doesn't find the lumps threatening either. "Nothing very interesting," he says to Nancy, who nods her clear understanding that everything is okay. She's been listening to doctors, interpreting their remarks, all of her child's life. Seashore doesn't think the lumps should be biopsied, just X-rayed. They should also be watched, to see if they're growing.

Rappeport says Brian also needs a chest X ray. He has a heart murmur, "seems to be the type that doesn't mean anything, but just to be sure." Nancy asks Rappeport if the X rays could hurt Brian, who received total body irradiation for his transplant.

No, says Rappeport. Since Brian's had the equivalent of 140,000 chest X rays, a couple more won't make any difference. Nancy says she thought the radiation Brian had received was the reason he shouldn't go out in the sun, and she assures Rappeport that despite his tan Brian always wears sunscreen. No, Rappeport says, "it isn't that," meaning that further radiation isn't the reason he fears the sun. He doesn't mention GVH or explain about Ricky Stott, but he gestures at Brian's tan and says, "Fine," indicating that his exposure to the sun is acceptable. "And he swims, under the water and everything," says Nancy. And he got straight A's, and wants to go to Notre Dame, and to be a football player *and* a baseball player.

"There's only one guy who can do that," says Rappeport. "Yeah, Bo Jackson," says Brian, who's both enthusiastic and composed. Being an only child, he's used to the company of adults.

Rappeport goes out to get a tape measure to calculate the size of the lumps and comes back with a fellow he wants to introduce to Brian. He goes out again for an order slip for the X rays, and returns with a colleague. When it's time to look down his throat,

Rappeport tells Brian to take his gum out. He protests; he's been blowing impressive bubbles.

"Your mother can hold it," Rappeport says, and Brian hands the gum to Nancy. Rappeport looks down his throat. "Tonsils," he says to Nancy, "that's good." Because tonsils are lymphoid tissue, their presence indicates the existence of an immune system. Brian lies on the table and Rappeport sits next to him, examining him. When Brian sits up, Rappeport stays beside him and, talking to Nancy, keeps his hand on the boy's shoulder, then on the side of his neck, the whole time.

"You can stop the Bactrim," he says to Nancy.

"I thought you told me it was forever," she says.

"You're right, because of the spleen."

Brian Murphy's splenectomy took place before he became Rappeport's patient. In any case, of course, a surgeon, rather than a hematologist, would have performed the operation, but Rappeport would have participated in the decision if Brian had then been in his care, and if that had been the case, he'd have remembered it now without prodding.

As Rappeport leaves the examining room, he's not exactly blushing but his complexion is darker than it normally is. "You ask about distance," he says. He shrugs, walking along. "I don't have any distance. It's the patients who make it who keep me going.

"How could one not be pleased? How could one not be? There are days when one's feeling down, and then something like this comes along. How could one not be pleased?"

Before Brian had his transplant, his eczema was so bad his hair stood straight up, stiff with the pus that came from his scratching-induced infections. His hands were red and raw. If he ate ketchup, his mouth burned from the acid. And, of course, without a bone marrow transplant, he was sure to die of infection or hemorrhage.

"Supposedly," Nancy said to me, "only males can get Wiskott-Aldrich. And females are carriers. They tell me it's a fifty-fifty chance if I have another boy he could have the same disease. I don't believe it."

Nancy has no Christopher Hough in her past and in her heart. Despite everything she's been through, she's loaded with joie de vivre. As she leaves, after Brian's clinic appointment, she says she thinks something may be wrong with her car; it was leaking fluid in the parking lot.

"Tell Mrs. Rap there'll be three more for dinner," says Nancy to Rappeport, on the way out the door with her mother and son. "Oh," she teases, "I forgot, you live here." At the hospital, she means.

"If anything's wrong," says Rappeport, referring to the possible car trouble, "call me."

"You're the only one I know here," says Nancy, not apparently conscious of the love and trust in her voice. "Who else would I call?"

FIVE

Uncertainty

"It's terrible to have leukemia," my sister Roberta said one day, her eyes closed, her tone sad, but as matter-of-fact as if she were discussing the grippe. Roberta's customary tone, on every subject, was outrage or hilarity or both. At another time, one of no particular physical torment, she said to me, "Madeline, this is misery." Again, she spoke without heat. She didn't need to; the depth of her horrible experience made the authenticity and authority of her commentary absolute.

Jennie Gossom, like Roberta, Wesley Fairfield, Peter Lariviere, and Rich Frisbee, had leukemia. The way in which it presented itself in Jennie, however, was more mysterious than in the other instances. The way it was understood was more equivocal, and the results of treatment—including the use of innovative technology against graft-versus-host disease—less predictable.

Jennie's transplant, in 1983, was the easiest part of her experience with leukemia. She has been free of the disease in the years since, and although she has some health problems that are almost certainly transplant-related, they are relatively minor: a lactose intolerance and, probably, developing cataracts.

Because her brother was her donor, she would have been likely to get the severe GVH more common in sex-mismatched transplants had the bone marrow she received not been T-cell-depleted. Anti-Leu 1, a monoclonal antibody designed to deplete T cells, was used for the first time in the course of Jennie's transplant. The graft-versus-host disease she had was so mild its existence was determined only by tests done on skin biopsies; the only symptom was a slight rash on her back. Despite T-cell depletion the graft from her brother took quickly, and her immune system reconstituted without trouble; the serious infections that were Rappeport and Smith's primary worry at the time of the experimentation on Jennie never materialized. Before new technology saved her, however, Jennie's suffering was extended and intense.

If down-to-earth Nancy Gossom were not the woman she is, Jennie would not now be alive. Jennie's mother is a nurse. Jennie says her mother's patients love her, that she offers counseling along with care. Nancy Gossom is sure of her judgments and not afraid to make them. When she talks about Jennie's symptoms and illness, and of her own fears, Nancy Gossom doesn't cry, nor does she inflect her voice in a way that either asks for or offers compassion. In conversation, she emphasizes her points with a lift of her eyebrows—heavy and dark, like Jennie's—and a definitive nod. Several times, she abruptly walks out of the room in which we're talking, sometimes to have a cigarette, sometimes just because she feels like it. As if stating the obvious, she says that at the announcement of bad news what you want is a drink. Jennie says it's her father who's the emotional one, "that's where we get it from," and Nancy doesn't seem soft, or sweet. She isn't sour, though, and she isn't hard. She is elastic; she finds out what she needs to know, and she is a woman of action. Jennie's illness can't have been the first bad time Nancy Gossom has lived through. Her manner is probably a result of both the success and scarring of her effort; she's clearly a seasoned meeter of tough challenges.

It was her opinion, when Jennie got sick, that her daughter was dying, but no doctor said so, and it was a long time—a year and a half—before anybody accurately named Jennie's disease. During that time Jennie steadily ran a fever, ranging around 102. She ached, all the time. Nevertheless, she went to work, although when she got home at the end of the day she sometimes sat shivering in her car, gathering enough strength to walk the few yards into her house. When she had her period, it went on and on, three weeks of steady heavy flow.

Jennie's body bruised easily. When she got home from her first hospital stay, in Gloucester, her mother helped her undress. "When I saw the purpura on her legs," Nancy Gossom says, "I almost passed out." Eighteen months later, a day before she was admitted to Boston's Brigham and Women's Hospital, Jennie's bleeding and bruising was so bad that "a lady at work asked me if I'd been in an automobile accident." But long before that, in the fall of 1981, her blood counts were consistent with her symptoms; her hematocrit was 7, against a normal count (for women; men have higher red counts) of 37 to 43.

It started in November, two months after Jennie turned twenty. She had graduated from high school, worked at a fast-food place, and then, just that past June, gotten a job as a secretary at Gorton's, a processor and distributor of frozen fish, a major employer in her city. Gloucester, an hour north of Boston, is a hilly, craggy New England coastal town that is still the home of a fishing fleet the Cardinal blesses every year. Jennie has lived in the town all her life. She grew up with her four older brothers and sisters in the cozy, small, pretty house in which she lives now, and virtually all her friends and family are nearby. "I don't take things for granted, like I used to," Jennie says now. "I know I still get mad at people, and things like that. I get frustrated. At things. But I just know, when I'm going up the highway and stuff and I look over the bridge at the trees and the foliage and stuff, it really sinks in how beautiful it is. I never knew that before. And the ocean. Things like that. Everyone says it, but it's true. You know? And I know how much I love my family. More than ever now."

First, she had a sore throat. "I just figured it was strep throat or something, and I don't think I even went to the doctor's. And then, around Thanksgiving, I started getting the achy joints and stuff. The backs of my knees and my ankles and stuff; it felt like arthritis. That's what brought me to the doctor's. Because I got to the point where I'd get up in the morning and I couldn't even bend over to iron or anything. So I went to the doctor, and he took a blood test, and they came back and told me my blood was low, and they thought maybe it was mono, so they really didn't do anything." The doctor's only suggestion was that she take a warm bath before going to work, in order to diminish the aching.

Jennie still felt terrible, though, so she went back to the doctor, but she says, "All they were doing really was just checking my blood, and then they thought maybe it was a mono hepatitis thing. They didn't seem to be really sure, and I was just feeling worse and worse and I just kept going back, and then my doctor referred me to a hematologist—the local hematologist. And they did more blood tests."

It was Christmastime. Nancy Gossom was sure it would be Jennie's last. Nancy had been reading up, and though no doctor had said so, was sure Jennie had leukemia. She kept her conviction to herself, but after the new year, she went with Jennie to the doctor and insisted they admit her to the hospital to find out exactly what was wrong. "And that's when I had my first bone marrow test done," says Jennie. It was so painful that the next time Jennie heard she had to have one, she says, "I just remember hollering out crying."

Rappeport makes very little of the pain bone marrow aspirations inflict. "It feels like pressure, that's all." Another hematologist has told me that the amount of pain a patient feels is directly related to the degree of disease he or she suffers. "When one aspirates a marrow packed with leukemia, it takes so much suction it hurts! But a remission marrow pulls easily—the patient has a brief, sharp pain." Nearly all the patients I talked to described the pain as excruciating; one or two said it wasn't too bad. To a certain extent, the degree of pain is supposed to be dependent on the experience and skill of the practitioner, but I've heard a patient scream and scream—only too audibly, through a closed door—when Rappeport's done an aspiration.

In the course of her treatment, Jennie had several bone marrow aspirations and about four bone marrow biopsies, which are even more painful. "Each time, it hurt more and more. It's like suction—it's like taking the suction out of a champagne bottle and just completely pulling it out. And it's just so painful." When Jennie was admitted to the Brigham, where she would eventually have her transplant, a doctor offered her morphine before a bone marrow aspiration, "and when they gave it to me, I remember it wasn't painful at all. And I felt like shaking someone, and saying, 'Why didn't someone tell me about this before?' "

For the first year and a half, the ordeal of the bone marrow tests was fruitless. "I think they were checking for anything like leukemia and things like that. Just trying to rule out everything they possibly could. All the serious things they were checking for were coming back negative. So that made us relieved." Her parents, she says, "practically cried with relief" when they first heard it wasn't leukemia. Nancy, however, wasn't relieved. Despite the reports she was hearing, Jennie had needed transfusions, and "I felt she was dying, but I kept it a secret." Instead, Nancy—who had insisted the local doctors do more—now asked that Jennie be transferred by ambulance to the Massachusetts General Hospital. "You don't demand, you ask," Nancy instructs.

Nancy was not happy with Jennie's care at the Mass General, and Jennie was miserable there, both physically and mentally. The Gossoms' experience was completely unlike the Fairfields' at the same hospital. Wesley and his family have only high praise for the skill, knowledge, and care he was given at the MGH, but the hematologist, says Nancy, "was aloof. He said twelve sentences the whole time. It was like pulling teeth." Different doctors came in at different times, instead of making rounds as a group, "so you had to go over it again, for each one." And still there was no diagnosis. "They thought it was maybe—different things," says Jennie. "They just could not put their finger on anything."

"They said it might be toxoplasmosis," says Nancy Gossom, "from the cat. We just could not get any answers."

Jennie had returned home and gone back to work, getting transfusions at the local hospital every two weeks. In April the hematologist Jennie had been seeing at the Mass General told her her spleen seemed to be malfunctioning and should be removed, but he didn't say exactly what was wrong.

In 1983 Dr. Stephen Emerson, who was a fellow at the Brigham—then Rappeport's hospital—was Jennie's doctor when she became an outpatient there six months after her stay at the Mass General. Like Diana Beardsley, he has a Ph.D. as well as an M.D., and like many doctors entering hematology today, he does most of his work in the laboratory. He says that Jennie's difficult-to-diagnose illness looked as if it was likely to be an autoimmune disease, such as lupus or juvenile rheumatoid arthritis, and so it would have been logical to remove her spleen, because the destruction of her cells—specifically, her platelets—would, in such diseases, have been taking place through an autoimmune mechanism mediated chiefly by the spleen. (In autoimmunity the body makes antibodies that destroy its own normal cells. In this case it would have been blood cells; specifically, red cells and platelets.) The other possibility likely to have struck doctors at this stage, he says, is that there was a malignancy in the spleen itself, and it would therefore be provident to remove it and find out.

The Gossoms were not privy to the reasoning Emerson assumes took place. "He thought," Jennie says, referring to her Mass General hematologist, "that at this point, you have to take the spleen out, because we have to try something. He told me that besides whatever was going on, I was pretty much in good health—they had done all the tests—and I shouldn't be in there more than seven days. But I ended up being in there three weeks. I lost about twenty pounds—I got down to less than ninety pounds." She could not eat; her vomiting and pain were intense.

The day after her spleen was removed, a doctor Jennie didn't know—a woman—walked into her room and asked her if she might be pregnant. "I was hoping I wasn't," Jennie says. "And I really thought in my mind that I wasn't, but everything was happening so quickly that I was just trying to—shrug it off. But at that point, when she came up to me and asked me, I knew that I very well could have been." Jennie had an abortion, on the doctor's advice and against her mother's—and her own—original wishes. "She was cruel," Jennie says of the doctor. "Not cruel, but—'You have to abort this!' I said, 'Wait a minute, I have to think about this.' "

Neither Rappeport nor Smith can point to a specific reason why Jennie had to have the abortion. They are not willing to criticize the other doctor's opinion, however, saying they weren't there and don't know the details of Jennie's condition at the time. Smith is willing to speculate: Maybe the doctors at the Mass General thought Jennie had PNH (paroxysmal nocturnal hemoglobinuria), a disease that destroys the patient's red cells. There are some similarities between PNH and the disease Jennie was ultimately found to have, and pregnancy usually kills patients with PNH. This diagnosis was considered, and ruled out, when Jennie was later evaluated at the Brigham. Smith thinks of another possible provocation for urging Jennie to abort. "In fact her platelet counts were bad, and therefore she was likely to get into trouble from bleeding into the placenta, or delivering a baby that wasn't normal. I guess it would make sense. But other than that, I don't know." When I suggest to Smith that the doctor might have given her advice on the basis of her own social prejudices—Jennie was young and unmarried—Smith doesn't disagree.

Despite the doctor's attitude and manner, however, Jennie did take some time to think. "I did a lot of soul-searching and stuff like that." In the hospital, she talked to a priest, who helped her; she doesn't feel guilty about her decision. "I just knew that at that point I had to look out for myself," a view the priest reinforced. She was also afraid that the treatment she'd had, particularly X rays, might have harmed the fetus. Her mother came to agree.

The result of the hospitalization, grueling as it had been, was positive. Despite all the pain she'd been suffering for over six months, and the mystery about its cause, her major emotion wasn't fright. "In a way," she says, she was frightened, "but in a way I wasn't, because they were doing all kinds of tests and they were coming back negative. That was making me feel better, but I think at this point I was more frustrated than anything. That I didn't know. And I was beginning to feel that people thought I was a hypochondriac. Because I'd go back to work and they'd say, 'What did the doctor say?' and I'd say, 'Well, they said everything— They still haven't found anything.' I was afraid they'd think I was just imagining these symptoms."

When Jennie got out of the hospital in May, "about Mother's Day," she says, "I was skinny as a rail and people were looking at me like 'What's the matter with you?' But at that point I was able to carry my own blood—I didn't have to have any more transfusions —so I felt better about that. Even though it wasn't the spleen, for some reason taking it out helped enough so that I didn't have to have any more transfusions. So that was May of '82, and I spent the rest of that year, going into '83, feeling pretty good, the best I had felt in a long time. I gained most of my weight back, probably fifteen pounds. And I felt pretty good. I took on a second job, I bought a new car, and I got a promotion.

"And then, in April of 1983, I started having small things wrong with me? Like I got—well, I shouldn't say small things. But I had a little pimple on my leg. It turned into a boil, and it was so bad that I couldn't even walk, and I had to go to the hospital, and they had to drain it. Things like that. I'd get a little cyst in my ear. And I just never put anything together, because I just didn't know what was happening."

Now, Jennie says, "I don't know much medicine or science, but I know a lot about red cells, white cells, and platelets."

Then, however, "I went to the doctors here and there for a few things, but they never seemed to know." But that summer, on a camping trip to Maine, her gums bled so profusely and steadily that someone asked her if she'd been eating licorice. (I once thought Roberta had lost some of her teeth, because they were so blackened with dried blood that they were obliterated.)

Jennie's period "would not stop. Still, I just wasn't concerned. I didn't even do anything when I came back that Monday. I went to work that whole week, and Friday I just really felt bad and run down, and I was still bleeding, so I called my doctor."

Jennie had been seeing Emerson at the Brigham since the previous January. She had changed hospitals and doctors, but her mother was endlessly looking for better care for her child. "Jennie was going down the tubes unless I did something," Nancy says. "I asked everybody if they knew somebody." One day she asked one of her own patients, a man who had written books about brain surgery and heart surgery, "You don't know a good hematologist, do you?"

" 'Matter of fact, I do,' " he said.

The name the man gave Jennie's mother was that of Dr. William Moloney, the doctor whose presence drew Rappeport to the Brigham. In 1983 Rappeport and a colleague were in charge of the Brigham's clinical hematology service. Jennie was never Moloney's patient. He had almost entirely retired from patient care by the time she got sick, but what Brian Smith identifies as "the Moloney philosophy—every patient's an individual"—still prevailed.

Nancy Gossom says she now tells everyone to go to the Brigham—for everything. Her generalization is too broad. No matter how famous the hospital, skill at diagnosis and cure and dedication to learning and care vary from department to department. One place might have the best neurosurgeons, for example, and others the best infectious disease specialists. In specialties with strong scientific appeal, there's another variable, invisible to patients: the quality and quantity of research, which determine the attractiveness of the department to house staff. In order to attract the best, opportunity for discovery and recognition have to exist. Hematology is a research-oriented specialty, and sophisticated, energetic experimentation is necessary to attract the brightest doctors, whose clinical expertise is in turn dependent on seeing many patients.

To make things more complicated, doctors in academic medicine move around a lot, so that hospital staffs—including the most senior people—vary from year to year. Neither Rappeport nor any of his closest associates now practice at the Brigham, for example, and although the hospital is one of several that make up the Harvard Medical School teaching, research, and health care facilities, where the amount of applied knowledge is staggering, the learning and caring of doctors and departments vary at the Brigham, as everywhere else.

The influence of a strong mentor, of course, is enormous and lasting. Emerson, now practicing academic hematology in Ann Arbor, Michigan, reveals this when he talks about presenting his understanding to the Gossoms, when Jennie first became a patient at the Brigham. He didn't know anything different from what doctors at the Mass General must have known, but his way of taking care of patients, he says, is to tell them what he's thinking—"it works better." I asked him if he'd learned this from Dr. Moloney and Rappeport. Yes, he said. It hadn't occurred to him until I asked, but those two men and David Rosenthal—the doctor with whom Rappeport then directed the hematology clinic—formed the way he practiced hematology.

Both the firm tone in which Emerson makes the statement and the fact that his realization came nearly a decade after the fact, and only after someone else pointed to it, indicate the way Rappeport, at least, exerts his influence. When doctoring (rather than medicine or science) is his subject, Rappeport teaches by example, and his students learn by osmosis. It is, like his relationships with his patients, more a family dynamic than a professional interchange. He is inarticulate about his own behavior and often apparently unaware of it. At his best, he inspires rather than instructs.

One morning in clinic a young woman, thin and bald and weak, sat on the edge of an examining table. Her transplant was still very recent; she'd been out of the hospital only a few weeks.

When Rappeport stepped out of the room, she said of his presence, not quite under her breath, "That will get me through the week." A nurse, sitting against the wall, was impassive. The words, just breathed out, were not for anyone in particular to hear. On another day, when Rappeport, making one of his several daily visits to his hospitalized patients, slouched into the room of a tall, muscular man, the patient demanded to know when he'd see him again. It was Rappeport's presence, said this man, that gave him life. Both these patients died, and the toll on Rappeport, especially of the loss of the young woman he'd transplanted, was heavy. But the reward of what he was able to do for them was great, also. Because he honored them during their worst times, they trusted him.

Roberta said that when she was undergoing her transplant, it was Rappeport's encouragement and that of the house officers that kept her going. She often felt so terrible she thought she was dying. "I never wanted to die, but there were plenty of times I thought I would [and the doctors would come by and] say I was doing great" and she believed them. Especially Rappeport, she said. Roberta saw him as a terrible pessimist—"downbeat" was her regular description—so "if he said things were okay, they were okay."

The Gossoms, particularly Nancy, recollect the switch to Rappeport's service as the beginning of good care and of hope for Jennie. When the Gossoms first went to the Brigham, Nancy told the staff that the family could deal with Jennie's fevers, that they "had become a way of life." A doctor patted her arm, indicating that that wasn't necessary, that there was something that could be done. Although Emerson maintains that Jennie's previous doctor must have harbored the same suspicions he did, he points out how his acknowledgment of them was a critical difference. "It's very unusual to find a patient who doesn't want to hear what you're thinking," he says. He told the Gossoms that Jennie might have aplastic anemia or one of the autoimmune diseases—juvenile rheumatoid arthritis, or lupus—she'd been told about, or she might have myelodysplasia, a word Jennie doesn't remember hearing. It is a condition Emerson defined as "preleukemic"—a term Jennie does recall. But in fact the reason Emerson gives for his good relationship with Jennie doesn't match hers. Jennie primarily remembers his kind manner, which for her included a *gentle* mention of hard facts. The Gossoms felt, from the beginning of their relationship with Rappeport's service, that the doctors there knew what they were doing—a feeling they gained, at least partly, from the detail in which Emerson revealed his thinking, even though the diagnosis was not definite for six more months.

It turned out that myelodysplasia was the disease from which Jennie suffered for eighteen months, but this became certain only retrospectively, when, in the summer of 1983, it transformed into leukemia. But in the six months that preceded the diagnosis, despite the fact that "preleukemia" was being discussed, Jennie says, "I just didn't worry about it. Because I didn't want to worry about it. It didn't really scare me, because it didn't sink in. And then I mentioned it to my parents, because they always came up to the doctor's with me, especially when I started going to Boston. And they didn't even seem to be concerned."

This "lack of concern" was in reality extremely good acting on the part of Gil and Nancy Gossom, both of whom were in fact terribly worried. Through the whole time of Jennie's illness, Nancy told Gil her fears. "Gil and I used to fight over this all the time. We—could—not—discuss—this—issue. I had to talk to my friends."

Although Jennie's symptoms may now seem to point clearly to myelodysplasia, there are several reasons why her case continued to stump Emerson, although he went over it with Moloney and Rappeport in 1983.

"She was a tough case," he says.

Jennie herself says, "I was just a real strange case."

Smith says some of the bone marrows were not of the best quality and it must have been hard to draw clear conclusions from them. Also, as Rappeport says, myelodysplasia tends to be seen in older people (Roberta had it at forty-eight), a point Smith and Emerson also cite; it's relatively rare for someone Jennie's age to have it. Then there is the fact that myelodysplasia isn't one condition but, like most of the diseases Rappeport deals with, a group of them. It's no wonder diagnosis is so difficult. The abnormality of the stem cell, he says, "results in abnormal production of all varieties of cells, either quantitatively and/or qualitatively. Rarely, on a genetic basis. Usually on an acquired basis. It's a very heterogeneous group of diseases." Sometimes, he says, there's a loss of material from chromosome 5.

Smith adds that there's chromosomal change in most people with myelodysplasia but the change is different from person to person. Though some have an abnormality of chromosome 5, for example, with other people it might be on chromosome 7. Some are translocations—a part of one chromosome changes places with a part of another—and some are losses. "A lot of those, actually, are losses of a whole chromosome." Smith goes on: "It's intriguing, but no one can say anything about it—for example, there's something called the 5q minus syndrome, which actually tends to go to acute leukemia less than some of the others, but the q just means the large arm. Chromosomes come with a large arm and a short arm. The large arm of chromosome 5 is missing." What's interesting about this, he explains, is that receptors for growth factors—substances that enhance cellular production—are at the same locus. "And that's just intriguing. You lose that, and then—something happens. Maybe that's pure coincidence. But if you could figure that out . . ."

"In essence," Rappeport says, myelodysplasia, like the more widely and intensely studied CML—chronic myelogenous leukemia—with its consistent chromosomal translocation, "is an unknown abnormality that starts in the stem cell and manifests itself in all the different cell lines."

Emerson says that Jennie was "unusual because although her counts were low, her platelets were large," another fact that made diagnosis difficult, and he explains too that it also meant bleeding wasn't a serious danger; the efficacy of platelets depends on overall surface, rather than on numbers. Adding to the confusion, says Emerson, was the fact that despite Jennie's low hematocrit she "was making a lot of cells. They were getting to the blood but being consumed quickly. That's unusual for leukemia." And finally, "She didn't have a lot of blasts."

Rappeport says that the delay in diagnosis made no difference in the outcome for Jennie, because the only way myelodysplasia can be cured is with a bone marrow transplant. This is because myelodysplasia—like chronic myelogenous leukemia—is a malignancy of the stem cell. Therefore, Rappeport says, myelodysplasia, like CML, is "going to be very important in terms of understanding the etiology of leukemias."

Smith explains further, showing the necessary connection between patient care and research. If someone with CML or myelodysplasia lives long enough, he says, that person will develop acute leukemia. With any particular patient it's impossible to say when, but over time the blood cells will change, and doctors can therefore watch the transition to acute leukemia take place; the blood drawn to monitor a patient's condition shows the cellular change in developing illness that acute leukemia, with its sudden onset, can't reveal. Because my sister's leukemia, like Jennie's, was preceded by myelodysplasia, I asked Rappeport if early transplantation, before one disease transformed into the other, was more likely to effect a cure. He told me—contradicting slightly the statement he made about late diagnosis not mattering with Jennie—that he couldn't be sure, because there were too few such cases to make the comparison and allow a clear evaluation, but that he thought yes, that early transplantation would be better.

In Jennie's case the question is moot, because her health was ultimately restored. But not before things got worse.

The first time I met him, Brian Smith sat in his laboratory office, a place distant from illness, where no patients come. Along with the medical books and journals and computer, there are novels—thrillers and science fiction—for hospital friends to borrow. There are tapes of Gregorian chant and Irish harp music and Handel and Vivaldi and one jazz tape called "This Is Ray Brown," a boom box on which to play them, photographs of classmates and mentors, cans of diet Coke (before he drinks from them, Smith wipes the tops with a tissue—"useless," he concedes, sticking to the habit anyway), and a variety of mementos, mostly jokes. He is a tall, big man in his late thirties, with curly brown hair and glasses. Despite the banter that makes up much of his personality, he looks, and is, deeply serious. "Leukemia," he said, "is a terrible disease." Making his statement to me, he looked straight ahead, at the wall, and spoke definitely and firmly and—somehow—threateningly.

In the summer of 1983, the week after that camping trip Jennie took with her family, she found she had leukemia. When she did call Emerson, she gave him her symptoms. "And he didn't say anything. And I said to him, 'Do you want me to wait until Monday to come up and see you?' And he must have known, because he said, 'No, I'd like you to come up this afternoon.' " Jennie's parents had gone shopping, but her father, knowing she would be calling the doctor, had told her to come and get him if she had to go to Boston. She picked him up at the local K Mart, "And—let's see— that was Friday afternoon, maybe around two or three o'clock? And the first thing Dr. Emerson did was take another bone marrow. And then we waited and waited—seemed like forever. And then he came back and he called us into his office."

This was significant. On her regular visits Jennie talked to Emerson in the examining room; the special place was a portent, to her, of a more serious discussion. "And he told me. He said, 'You know, for a long time you haven't been feeling good.' He goes, 'Well, there's some leukemia blasts in your blood.' " "Blast" is a suffix that denotes a stage of immaturity and sometimes a lack of differentiation in most blood cells. Megakaryoblasts precede megakaryocytes and then thrombocytes, in development. Some myeloblasts become neutrophils, others eosinophils, others mast cells. Despite their identical appearance at this point, however, each of these myeloblasts is part of a "committed" cell line. That is, by this stage of development, their ultimate form and function are determined; they will not divide into other sets of cells. In fact, their normal destiny, like that of other blood cells, has been formed several stages back. "A blast in peripheral blood," says Rappeport, "means something's abnormal. But if I look in bone marrow and see blasts, and they look normal, that's okay."

Emerson says he saw "pathoblasts in the marrow." You can tell a blast in the marrow is abnormal, Rappeport says, "morphologically. By the size and shape, and characteristics of the nucleus, with lymphoblasts having somewhat different characteristics than myeloblasts."

The sight of malformed blasts was confirmation of Emerson's fears for Jennie. The fact that he decided to do a bone marrow was itself threatening; at least in Rappeport's circle, well-prepared blood samples tell most of what needs to be known. (For diseases less horrifying than the ones he tends to treat, examination of the bone marrow isn't as strong a signal of disaster. "You might do a marrow in severe iron deficiency to assess the iron stores," Rappeport says, offering examples, "or you might do one in a person with an abnormal protein to look for lymphoma, and it might be benign." He adds a snide remark about some doctors doing the relatively expensive test for the money.) In the four years I spent watching Rappeport, I saw diagnostic marrows done only with a strong and highly educated suspicion of bad trouble, virtually always confirmed—as it was for Jennie, eighteen months after her symptoms first appeared.

The discharge summary that describes the details and results of Jennie's first long stay at the Brigham includes the history of her illness and a report on the means of diagnosis:

ADMISSION LABORATORY DATA: Hematocrit 26.2. White count 10.6; 22 polymorphonuclear cells, 18 bands, 19 lymphocytes, 4 monocytes, 7 metamyelocytes, 5 myelocytes, 6 promyelocytes, 19 blasts. Platelet count 9,000. Peripheral blood also showed 200 nucleated red blood cells. Smear was remarkable for large amounts of nucleated red blood cells, large numbers, 10–20 percent blasts, with dark cytoplasm, rare nucleolus, slightly clumped chromatin and immature myeloid forms and decreased platelets. The bone marrow aspirate showed a preponderance of blasts, as noted above, with dark cytoplasm, slightly clumped chromatin and rare nucleoli. There were decreased megakaryocytes and normal erythroid precursors. Her bone marrow was sent for chromosome studies and surface markers.

The report from the cytogenetics laboratory said Jennie had extra copies of chromosome 8. And, "In the 10 cells with the extra #8 and fewer than 47 chromosomes, chromosome loss was random." It cites the frequency with which this particular change occurs in the specific leukemia subtype Jennie had.

"Most leukemics have chromosomal change," Smith says. "You go back fifteen years, we used to say that was true in 15 percent of acute leukemias. Then there were better techniques, and we said 50 percent. Then we get even better techniques, and we say 85 percent. So it's likely that virtually all of them have it."

Before that much detail was obtainable on Jennie, however, the diagnosis was made:

> ASSESSMENT ON ADMISSION: The patient was felt to have an acute leukemia with an atypical presentation after a 1½ year illness characterized by peripheral destruction of all cell lines and fevers. This has now clearly evolved into an acute leukemia with a preponderance of blasts in the bone marrow.

"I think," Jennie says, speaking of that August day when Emerson told her she had leukemia, "if they didn't find a diagnosis, I would have probably died from depression at that point. Because just not knowing is sometimes worse than anything."

All the same, and with it all behind her, Jennie still cried at the telling. "I just looked at my father and—he just turned white as a ghost, and it was like I was in a different world at that point, you know?" It's the same world that Wesley Fairfield and Peter Lariviere and Ricky Stott and Rich Frisbee have inhabited. "Like everybody says—why me?" says Jennie. "At twenty years old I thought I should have been at the prime of my life, getting ready to maybe get married, or something. I had gone out with someone for six years, and things weren't going *great*, but I just felt like it should have been one of the happiest times of my life."

The first person she thought of, though, was not herself. "I looked at my father, and I said, What's he going to do if anything happens to me? I have two sisters and two brothers, but I'm the baby. And he's always—even now—he smothers me, you know? He's so emotional." The day Jennie's disease was finally identified as leukemia, Gil Gossom was too overcome to tell the rest of the family. Jennie made the necessary calls. At a later time, talking about her father, Jennie says how much she values her father's emotional personality. When he talked to me, Gil Gossom *sobbed* recollecting Jennie's illness, becoming inarticulate after a few sentences. "I respect my father for crying," Jennie says.

Gil Gossom is short and heavyset. "A prime candidate for a heart attack," says Rappeport, who says he worried "the whole time" that Jennie's father would have one.

"He used to point at him," Nancy Gossom says, using a quick imitative gesture, "and say, 'You're going to have a heart attack.' " She's exasperated. "He should have said the opposite. He should have told him he's *not* going to have a heart attack."

The tactlessness, and his obliviousness to it, is typical of Rappeport. He was stating the facts as he saw them, the worry that was on his mind. Some of his other remarks lack the concern that makes them excusable. "He told my sister she talked too much," Jennie says.

When Jennie's myelodysplasia transformed into leukemia, she became a potential patient of Rappeport's. Because myelodysplasia is a stem cell disease, the leukemia that evolves from it also afflicts the most basic blood cell. Some leukemias, because they originate farther along in hematopoietic development, can be cured with the use of chemotherapy alone. In these instances it is possible to kill the cells where malignancy originates and still leave regenerative function. Wesley Fairfield's leukemia was such a disease. Although a bone marrow transplant was his best chance at cure, it was not his only one.

The same was not true of Jennie. Only therapy that included eradication of the stem cell could work in the long term, for her. Although she, like Wesley, had AML, the knowledge that she had had myelodysplasia was critical because it *dictated* bone marrow transplantation. But first, as with Wesley—and with Peter Lariviere and Rich Frisbee—there was the grueling ordeal of chemotherapy designed to achieve the remission necessary for the bone marrow transplant's optimal chance at success.

Right after he told Jennie she had leukemia, Emerson put her in the hospital.

"I still remember the day I was admitted," says Jennie, "because it was my niece's first birthday. It was August 12, 1983. And I didn't get out until a week before Halloween." First, there was the family to tell. "So this was like six o'clock by now," Jennie says. "It was a very long afternoon. They admitted me, and my mother and my brother came up that night. And that was a hard point—just seeing everybody for the first time, after finding out and everything. What do you say to people? What do people say to you? It's not just another day anymore. It's just how it's going to be."

Nancy Gossom, her fears confirmed, found the right words. Her daughter quotes her: " 'Jennie,' she said, 'I know how bad it sounds, but we've been a year and a half now trying to find out what's the matter with you, and as serious as it is, at least they know what it is now, and they can try to work on it.' And I knew she was right," Jennie says. "That's when they really started."

"She had an extraordinarily difficult, prolonged hospitalization," Rappeport says. "Which went on for *months*. With fever, and her counts weren't coming back, and things like that—in part because of the myelodysplastic syndrome, with which the recovery of the counts is usually much, much slower." Doctors were trying to get the disease to revert to myelodysplasia. "With leukemia secondary to myelodysplasia, that's the best you're going to come to," says Rappeport.

It was a ten-week period of misery and terror, much of which Jennie doesn't remember, because of the painkilling and antinausea drugs she received. She was admitted with an abscess on her vulva and developed one on her buttock. "They couldn't operate on it for three months," Nancy Gossom says, because Jennie lacked granulocytes to fight infection, primarily as a result of the leukemia rather than of the treatment for it. "I thought she was never going to have white cells again." Jennie developed hemorrhoids so painful she needed morphine in order to move her bowels. She frequently had high fevers. She suffered all the vomiting and diarrhea common to people undergoing chemotherapy, and she minded terribly the loss of her long brown hair. "I always tried to say, Well, it could be worse; it will grow back. But I felt like, I wish I had a husband at this point. I wish I had my life all settled."

"They gave me something that kind of takes away the nausea and stuff," Jennie says. "It's a continuous drip. That helped a lot, but I was pretty much out of it a lot of the time. And then I did get to feeling a little better, and I started getting short-winded. And then they told me that that could be congestive heart failure, so they put me down in intensive care. Everything was urgent. Something that could be little to anybody else, I noticed that they were right on top of it, and taking care of things right away."

Jennie's problem was pulmonary edema, fluid in the lungs. Nancy Gossom says she was the first to notice that Jennie was restless and short of breath, and that she called it to the doctors' attention, along with her observation that Jennie was "filling up with fluid." "I was always glad that my mother was a nurse," Jennie says, "because I had my own private nurse." Jennie was in the ICU overnight, and Gil remembers that a resident stayed for thirty-six hours, but Jennie says the experience was "scary. That was really scary. Very depressing. Everything was serious. And I still remember—there was a male nurse up there, and he came in to see me, and he asked me if I was afraid to die." Out of all she has to tell, Jennie is uniquely bewildered by this blow.

Brian Smith remembers that as a beginning doctor he was once sent, while on a psychiatry rotation, to see a terminally ill woman. "And when I got back, they asked me how she felt about dying. 'Like hell, I imagine,' I said. 'But I didn't feel I knew her well enough to ask.' " No such sense of decency restrained Jennie's nurse. "I could not believe that he was asking me that. And the only thing I remember saying to him was, 'Aren't you?' "

Lugubriousness was bad, but Jennie didn't like the other end of the scale either, nurses who were "chipper and cheery. After, it was fine, but you get mad when everyone else is healthy and you're sick," she says.

Emerson refers to this period as "a very long nadir" and praises Jennie, years later, for her courage, for her determination to live, for her cooperation in her care. For managing to eat. "People sometimes *die* from not eating." "Jennie never complained," Nancy Gossom says, but Jennie remembers it differently. She praises Emerson, who came and sat by her bed, at this time and later, too—when he was no longer her doctor but remained her friend—and held her hand as she cried. "I never expected to have a doctor who was a friend."

Finally, on October 26, Jennie left the hospital; her counts were beginning to come back but were still so depleted that she was scheduled for a platelet transfusion three days later.

"And then they didn't want to waste much time with the bone marrow transplant. I didn't either—because I felt that the longer I wait the more chances that I could relapse before it happens, and I don't want to give myself the first chance of relapse. I'd like to be in remission, you know?"

Rappeport says remission is impossible to achieve in leukemics whose disease has derived from myelodysplasia, and Jennie's condition was now "the best you can hope for," the goal of the first chemotherapeutic induction. She had reverted to her preleukemic state.

"In acute leukemia," Smith says, "the kind where you have abnormal cells and normal cells, you knock out the abnormal cells. They take forever to come back, thank goodness, but the normal cells come back with a vengeance. Still, if your whole stem cell's bad, all you've got is bad stuff to come back. Slightly *better* stuff may come back, and we see that all the time. Even though it's a stem-cell disease, you get back not leukemia-looking cells but preleukemic cells, after chemotherapy. Why does that happen? I haven't the foggiest idea. Nobody knows. It's interesting. You're differentiating the cells somehow. You're making them better with chemotherapy," rather than simply eliminating them. "You'd like to be able to figure it out."

This is the leitmotif that constantly plays for Rappeport and Smith. The hope of solving the problem—the "conundrum," Rappeport calls it—of terrible disease through discovery is half of the "fun" they say is inherent in their work. The other half is the active nature of bone marrow transplantation. Despite the uncertainty of its outcome, the decision to try it has high definition: Disease will go and health will return. There's nothing palliative about the attempt; an absolute is the goal. Though they take good care of people who die, they do not see their mission as the cure of dying people.

Smith agrees that the reason Jennie's first hospitalization was so long was that she had a stem-cell disease. The problem was so fundamental to the production of all the hematopoietic and immune system cells that the return of even imperfect function was slower than usual. Having attributed the difficulty to myelodysplasia, however, he immediately expands, equivocates, and speculates. It's possible, too, that Jennie had a problem with DNA repair, a lessened ability to reconstitute *any* damaged cells. "If there's an intrinsic problem in what you were born with, what you got from Mom and Dad, then you might expect more toxicity," Smith says. There are people, he goes on, who, when they go out in the sun, "get skin tumors all over the place," not because the sun damaged their skin more than anyone else's, "but because they can't fix it." So with the kind of response Jennie had to chemotherapy, "there may be something intrinsically wrong that we're just unable to figure out yet."

The problem might go beyond even the stem cell. "It might be the stroma," the support for the bone marrow, the network on which the bone marrow grows. It's "that portion of the bone marrow that doesn't come from the bone marrow stem cells. It comes from other things; it's more the same kind of cells that your blood vessels or your skin is derived from. All kinds of big, juicy cells. There's extracellular matrix and that makes a glue on top of it, which is somehow important for telling cells where they're supposed to go, and how they're supposed to grow, and how they're supposed to connect to one another." If the stroma in Jennie's bone marrow was defective—"if she had bad soil, if she had bad bone marrow microenvironment, if she had a bad ditch for the bone marrow to grow in—all favorite terms of hematologists—that would cause a delay in the recovery of her blood-making cells."

But if that were the case, the transplant itself should have taken a long time to work, "because all you can transplant is the stem cell. You don't really transplant the stroma, the basis on which it grows. Therefore, if that's bad, you'd expect that somebody else's bone marrow would take a while to grow also." But this didn't happen with Jennie; despite the predictive elements that said her great danger in undergoing a transplant would be graft failure, this was not the case. The transplant itself—despite scares for the doctors and misery for Jennie—went smoothly and easily. For a bone marrow transplant.

But first, there was further preparation. She had to have her wisdom teeth out. Exhaustive dental work, a safeguard against infection, is commonplace before bone marrow transplants. "They treat you like an astronaut," Roberta said. And then Jennie went into the hospital for surgery, to have shunts placed. "I went in, and when I came out of the anesthesia, I had bandages on this arm here"—she holds out her right arm—"but there was no shunt in it. And in the left arm there was a shunt, because I guess they had failed on one arm. That's what these marks are for." She shows her scars. "And this arm," the left one, where the shunt had been left in place, "I could not move. It turned out that that one had failed, too. So they had to put me back into surgery again. And they took the shunt out of my arm, and when I woke up again from surgery, I had the shunt in my leg. So I had two scars from the shunts that didn't even work, but this one, thank God, it worked, and it stayed in until after the bone marrow transplant. And I still had the Hickman in.

"And then I got to have maybe two weeks at home with my family. I was home for Thanksgiving, and I went back the first week in December."

Before Jennie underwent the transplant that would return her health she had one more particularly harrowing incident to endure: She had to hear about the transplant before it happened.

Up until this point, Rappeport's involvement with Jennie and her family had been what he calls "peripheral." The Gossoms say Rappeport mentioned a transplant as actually "being in the works" before they fully realized it was even an option. This juxtaposition creates a quandary common to people who do not know Rappeport well and who do not spend a great deal of continuous time with him. He often seems oblivious to the fact that anyone not present during a conversation or action—and sometimes even a thought—can't know it unless they're told; the best the absentee gets is an impatient, usually partial, allusion to the missed information.

"I didn't like him," Jennie says of the beginning of her relationship with Rappeport. "Nobody in my family liked him. But my mother said, 'Jennie, he's a very knowledgeable doctor.' " Nancy said, "We're not buying his personality." Neither Gil nor Nancy wanted Jennie to know how bad things were, but Rappeport said she had to know. "It all came out," says Nancy, "that son of a gun!"

Between her chemotherapy hospitalization and the transplant, the two-week period during which Jennie, regularly transfused, was having shunts put in and her wisdom teeth taken out, "we did have the consultation with Dr. Rappeport, too. And he had to go over *everything* with us. What was going to happen and stuff like that. And then he told me, 'Jennie, this is 1983. If this were 1985, your chances would probably be better, because we would know more. Now there's a fifty-fifty chance.' He just came right out and said it. And that's one problem I had with Dr. Rappeport—he said what was on his mind, and he laid the cards on the table. And I just felt like sometimes he could've used a little discretion, but he didn't.

"I had to let that sink in. I go, 'You mean, there's a fifty-fifty chance that I could die?' And he goes, 'Yes.' And that kind of—that was my first real breakdown. And it took a while to sink in, that I could go in the hospital and not come out again."

During this conversation Jennie found out she'd be sterile. "I would love to have kids," she says. "It's something that I've always looked forward to. But if I don't live, I'm not going to have kids. But it took a while. It took a couple of years. Even now [seven years later] it still bothers me off and on. Like my sisters and brothers all have kids. And it's like, you realize now, when parents talk about their kids, you say"—as she quotes her own thoughts, Jennie's voice shakes—"Well, I'm probably never going to be able to talk like that. Unless I adopt someday. So I think of those possibilities, that maybe I'll be able to adopt. And I think I've accepted it. Pretty much. I know there's nothing else I can do about it."

"Jennie's sterile," Nancy Gossom says. She gives a quick, fierce nod. "That was something else to deal with."

At the informed-consent meeting, Gil says, "I was scared. But after that, I always felt better after I talked to Dr. Rappeport." It could be Scott Fairfield speaking, though Gil is forty years older than Scott, a father rather than a brother, and unlike the younger man in experience, personality, or temperament. Jennie and her mother, however—despite the years that have passed, their gratitude, and their full acknowledgment of Rappeport's expertise—still think he should have acted differently. "I didn't want to be a number," Jennie says. "I wanted some friendliness."

The beginning of her hospitalization for the transplant was a time of emotional as well as physical isolation for Jennie. The purification of her system and environment, each detail performed for good medical and scientific reasons, nevertheless sounds ritualistic. "I remember distinctly the day I had to go into the bone marrow room [the laminar flow room]," says Jennie. "I had to have a shower and completely sterilize myself. They gave me about twenty face cloths, and I'd put a little Betadine on one face cloth and do my face. Then I'd have to take another face cloth and do another part of my body, and I could never use the face cloth twice on the same part of the body—or on a different part of the body. Once all that was done, they gave me sterile towels and I dried myself off. Then they gave me a johnny and slippers, and they put me in the wheelchair, and they wrapped sheets around me. They didn't even want me breathing in the air out in the hallway, so they covered me up completely, even my face. And they wheeled me over to the room. And that was traumatic."

Louise Lariviere, Peter's mother, saw him similarly draped—when he was on his way to receive radiation—and counts it as one of her worst moments: "To see your child like that," a body covered with a sheet, and to reasonably see the image as a foreshadowing, was terrible indeed. Ernie and Louise Lariviere left the decision as to whether or not to have a transplant to Peter—at sixteen, says Louise, he was old enough to choose. Martha and Ed Fairfield felt the same about Wesley, at nineteen. And Nancy Gossom refers to Jennie as "grown up" at the time of her illness. She was twenty-two when she had her transplant and an open, sensitive person.

Talking to me on the telephone many months after her transplant, Roberta apologized for complaining. I remonstrated with her: Who had more right to complain? At this stage her physical condition was terrible; she was able to do very little for herself. I did not think she would live much longer. "With all you've been through," I said. "No, Madeline," she said, correcting me with her sad, sure tone. "All I have now is my dignity."

Jennie too talks about being sick "with dignity," and her voice slows at the word, every consonant of which she carefully sounds.

In Jennie's telling, the transplant hospitalization was at first frightening and then sometimes sickening—like everyone else, she especially cites the disgusting-tasting, intensely nauseating bowel prep—but mostly, after a while, it was boring. She kept busy, she says, watching soap operas. "Seeing other people's problems," she says, "kept me from going stir-crazy." And crocheting an afghan. "They sterilized the yarn."

Her boyfriend was steadfast, as he had been throughout. They had gone together from their early teens, and although their relationship before Jennie got sick had become rocky, he proposed to her when she was in the hospital. "I'm not saying it was all sympathy," Jennie says, "but it was something he wouldn't have done at that point, if I wasn't sick. But I couldn't say anything. I just took it in stride, and I took the ring and everything. And it was a good year and a half, two years later that we realized that it just wasn't going to work out. And I knew it all along. It had nothing to do with the illness. He loved me, I know that, and I loved him, but we just weren't meant to be together. And I felt fine, because I know he didn't leave me because of my illness." Once she was well, though, "One of the problems was dating people. I didn't want to have to tell them what was wrong—what had happened to me, that I had leukemia. I don't know why, but I was just embarrassed to go into the details. Maybe I figured that they wouldn't want me. 'I don't want somebody who's had leukemia.' Or maybe they'd think it was contagious or something. It just really bothered me. I dated a few guys, and when it got to the point that maybe the relationship was going to get close, I'd back off.

"But Jay [her current boyfriend] had gone out with my cousin for a long time, and he already knew. He was the first one that I really felt comfortable with, and I talked to him about everything. And he accepted everything and was fine. When it came time to talk to him about birth control and stuff I said—well, that bothered me, to tell him that I was sterile. We talked a long time, and he got it out of me. And he seemed to accept it. That was a big turning point, to get through that obstacle with him. I knew down the road if anything was going to become of this relationship I would have to tell him that I would never be able to have any kids, and I was afraid that he wouldn't accept it. But I was really glad that I got involved with him, and he knew what was the matter with me, and he wanted me even after he knew what was the matter with me."

During the hospitalization Jennie's family were, as ever, constant. Her parents brought the food she liked: lobster pies, chowder, pork chops with rice. Some of it survived the sterilizing procedure, although "hard candy melts." Her father baked sugar cookies for her and called at six-thirty in the morning, waking her but reassuring himself that she was all right. Jennie's employer held her job for her, and every day someone from work called or sent a card or both. Her boyfriend's sister, a nurse at a nearby hospital, came over at lunchtime every day, and with the overwhelming exception of terrible illness, Jennie lived in a kind world. She began to like Rappeport. "I just accepted the type of person he was. I had to. I knew he couldn't really be like Dr. Emerson, holding my hand and saying everything's okay, and things like that. But he was a person I could talk to. I just knew he was a blunt person. And once in a while he'd have his bad days, and everybody would know it."

The crowds of doctors coming in, Gil says, "in their long coats, scared me. I wouldn't have been scared if they seemed like individuals." He became adept at tracking Rappeport down, and he always got an answer that satisfied him. "He gives you enough to digest each day."

Rappeport says the hospitalization is the time he gets to know the patients and becomes close to them. Jennie says that when she was in the hospital, Rappeport got friendlier, "more human," coming by and joking with her.

Rappeport characterizes Jennie's stay as "a benign course." It lasted from December 16, 1983, to February 21, 1984, which was, especially for the time, relatively brief. She had no complications, and her counts came back quickly. This was surprising not only because of the suppositions Smith posits about stem-cell disease and stroma, but because T-cell depletion of the marrow is known now, and was known then, to frequently delay or even prevent bone marrow engraftment.

Jennie's transplant took place two years after Peter Lariviere's and almost a decade after Ricky Stott's. At this point Rappeport knew far more than he wanted to about the devastation of GVH, but he had also learned that older people and people whose donor is of the opposite sex are most likely to get it—"prognostic features that were not a universally accepted opinion at the time"—and that removing mature T cells from the marrow has a reasonable likelihood of preventing GVH or of mitigating its intensity.

There is no sure way to predict the occurrence or severity of graft-versus-host disease; neither Peter Lariviere nor Ricky Stott were considered to be at high risk at the time of their transplants, nor would they be now. Jennie, however, was in one of the two high-risk groups, because her donor was the older of her two brothers—Gilbert Gossom, Jr., whom she and her parents call Gilly. In a picture taken a year after the transplant, at Christmastime, Gilly and Jennie stand in front of the tree, under a red paper bell. Jennie's hair has grown in in a lighter color than it was before the transplant; it matches Gilly's now. Since the time the picture was taken, Jennie has developed pollen allergies that she had never had before, but her brother had. "We did that," Smith says, looking and sounding pleased. It's another interesting knot to appraise in straightening out the immune system's tangle. Peter Lariviere apparently got his brother's sinus trouble along with Gary's bone marrow, and Smith talks about another patient who "six or seven months after the transplant has suddenly discovered he can't eat peanut butter," to which his donor has been allergic all along. The patient "itches like crazy when he eats peanut butter now. So we do this regularly.

"It's very interesting. An allergy is basically your immune system overreacting to something it wants to get rid of. The whole purpose of your immune system is to go around and find invaders and kill them off. But a second thing it does, it remembers when it's killed them off and what it's seen before. That's why vaccination works. The reason we shoot up children with DPT and so forth is not that your kid is incapable of mounting an immune response to those things—those of us who never got mumps, measles, rubella vaccine but got the disease, we were okay. We were sick for a while, but we were okay. And in the days of the polio epidemic, not everybody died of paralytic polio. In fact, most people who got polio probably just had diarrhea. But some people died from it.

"We're all capable of making an immune response. The reason vaccination works is because if you've done something once, your immune system remembers it, and it does it much faster and much better the second time." And this works, even if the disease has been killed when it enters your system. "Your immune system reacts against it; it actually tries to kill the killed stuff, but it doesn't matter, because it's already dead, and then when you see it again, you react to it lickety-split. And never give it a chance to give you paralytic polio. Or whatever the disease is."

In the case of allergies, "the memory can be carried over from one person to another." It could be in the B cells or the T cells, or "it could even come all the way from the stem cell. Because whatever allowed the person to make an allergy in the first place could have been either of two things. Either the immune system is intrinsically—genetically—abnormal and always creates too vigorous a response (manifest as allergy to, say, peanut butter) or the immune system is intrinsically okay but sometime during its initial exposure to peanut butter the response went awry, just once, and that one mistake is then carried along for life. If the latter explanation is true, then the T-cell depletion might deplete the cells with the memory of peanut butter and on reexposure, all would go well the next time around. But if the former explanation is true," if there's a basic genetic overreaction, "then even if you didn't carry over the cells with memory, reexposure to peanut butter would again result in allergy. Because it would be *intrinsic* to your immune system.

"The ability of some people to make a better immune response to a particular foreign invader probably relates to HLA type. You know," says Smith, as he starts explaining HLA using almost exactly the same words Rappeport does, "it couldn't just be there so it would mess up our chances of transplanting people. I mean, it could be. Life could be that perverse. But I don't really think so. There's got to be some other reason for it." Part of the reason has to do with the individual variations in the immune response, according to Smith, with how well the person makes an immune response. "That presumably is what allows some people to survive the plague." Frank Grosveld made a similar point to me in explaining that one way or another, AIDS would eventually lose its virulence. "Everybody's immune system is slightly different," Smith says, "and even if you have something that kills 90 percent of people, 10 percent of people have an immune system that deals with it just fine, thank you, and survive and go on and make the next generation. So presumably part of the reason for having a huge diversity of immune systems, the ability to respond to it, is that on a population basis it saves the species. There may be a million and one other reasons for doing it as well, but that's one reason. That's the long way around of saying why you can get your brother's or sister's allergies.

"How your immune system works," says Smith, talking even faster than usual because he's due to make rounds ("I'll try to do this in three minutes," he says), "is by wandering around in your body and looking at everything it can find and trying to tell whether it belongs to itself or to something else. And if it finds something that belongs to something else, it kills it off. That's how it knows to kill germs. Viruses. And, probably, in part, how it knows to kill tumor cells. It's possible that all of us are getting little tumors all the time, and our immune system is killing these tumors as it goes along, as it wanders throughout the body. How does it know that something doesn't belong to you? That's a complicated story. One way it knows is by HLA, which is why you have to be an HLA-identical brother or sister, in general, to get a transplant accepted. Except in experimental circumstances.

"To reject a graft, not have it grow— Let's say I'm the person getting the bone marrow transplant. My immune system sees your cells coming in and says, Whoa, they don't belong here, I'm going to get rid of them. That's graft rejection. Graft-versus-host disease is, I'm sitting there, my immune system's been taken away by radiation or whatever, your cells come in. Where does your immune system come from? Straight out of your bone marrow. Therefore, we're not dealing with a single immune system, which is what you're dealing with in a kidney transplant or a heart transplant, or a pancreas transplant. In a bone marrow transplant we have two immune systems playing the game. One of them is the recipient's—host's—immune system. The other one is the donor's immune system. So your immune system comes in, looks around at me, and does exactly what it's supposed to be doing in you. Which is, it starts wandering around, tries to figure out what belongs there, and all of a sudden says, Whoops! *None* of this belongs here. Now, why it picks the skin and the liver and the gut to attack, and not the kidneys and the nose, and who knows what else in there—I don't know."

In any case, "the relevant part of the immune system here happens to be the T lymphocytes." By the time of Jennie's transplant, T-cell depletion had been tried. Smith and Rappeport decided to use a new agent—anti-Leu 1—in this instance, for two reasons. The first was an effort to look for a better method than those they had already used. Rappeport says that there are some "theoretical problems" with the first monoclonal antibody he tried, "but in fact we weren't doing it in the right kind of patient." He had then switched to a second monoclonal antibody, one that had been tried on ten or twelve people. It was "okay, but not perfect"; one patient, at least, developed chronic GVH. More problematically—and more revealing of the frustrations in Rappeport's life—interlaboratory and administration power plays made the use and appraisal of the method too difficult to be worth further effort. "Anytime anything went wrong, it was either, one, we did not know how to diagnose GVH or, two, we had not done the processing right. Or whatever." In addition, the intense battle going on between the doctor manufacturing the substance at a neighboring hospital and a doctor highly placed at Rappeport's hospital "led to our feeling that this was just totally inappropriate and could not continue."

The drug company that made anti-Leu 1 was then initiating clinical trials of the substance. Rappeport and Smith enrolled Jennie in the study, thus making her transplant experimental and subject to outside review, both by the hospital's Human Subjects Committee and by the federal government. The FDA was involved simply because the manufacturer of anti-Leu 1 was in another state. "I can shoot this wastebasket into you if it doesn't cross state lines," Rappeport says. Smith says that in general, dealing with a company is better than working with a doctor producing a substance in his own laboratory, because the company, doing business across the country and around the world, has to adhere to FDA regulations. Only trust protects a private arrangement.

Anti-Leu 1, Rappeport says, appeared to fulfill the necessary criteria. In addition to binding to rabbit complement and recognizing and destroying mature T cells, it "did not go back and recognize *very* immature T cells, which we did not want it to do." If it had, the immune system, lacking any cells with which to reconstitute itself, would have been unable to do so. Also, its attack was restricted to cells of the immune system, those descended from the lymphoid stem cell. "A series of studies showed it did not appear to have an effect on the hematopoietic stem cell."

With Jennie, who is proud of having been the first person on whom anti-Leu 1 was used, the monoclonal antibody was apparently effective, although in fact it is impossible to know for sure. It is true, however, that she not only escaped serious GVH but also was spared the terrible consequences that can accompany T-cell depletion. With T-cell depletion "There's a greater incidence of returning malignancy and of lymphoproliferative disorders," says Rappeport, "but that may be because patients you might have lost from severe GVH may be living, and so there might be a higher at-risk population."

Jennie did not develop serious infections after the transplant, nor was she afflicted with a subsequent lymphoma, a terrifying possibility that has afflicted other patients of Rappeport's: One posttransplant man seemed to be free of malignancy in the morning, developed disease apparently within hours, and died from rapidly proliferating tumors less than a week later. But there is no way of knowing if Jennie would have escaped these devastating trials anyway. Her prompt engraftment in the face of the probability that either myelodysplasia or T-cell depletion, let alone both, would *increase* graft rejection is simply inexplicable.

There were fruits from the research done on Jennie, ranging from calculating dosages to understanding the normal proliferation of B cells. "When we started to watch her," Smith says, referring to examining Jennie's blood cells after the transplant, "she came back initially with a lot of B cells, not T cells. And they happened to be a particular kind of B cell—that is, the kind of B cell that people with chronic lymphocytic leukemia have. And they were *all* B cells that looked like chronic lymphocytic leukemia. All of them. That scared us; that was not supposed to be present in normal people. So we said, 'This is not good. This is some terrible thing that we have done here.' But it turned out that in other ways they were not like the cells of chronic lymphocytic leukemia. And then we started to look at people who didn't get GVH—they didn't have T cells removed, they were just people who didn't get GVH. And they came back with the same odd-looking cells, all the time. And then we got better at looking at these things, and we looked in you and me, and we realized they were a normal component." Smith looked to see where the cells came from—whether they were Jennie's original ones or the donor's, whether they descended from the same or a different progenitor. "Fortunately they turned out to come from different cells." None of this worry or the details of the research were transmitted directly to the Gossoms, but they heard, all along, snatches of the work going on that reassured them. "It was, 'Brian says this,' or 'Brian says that,' " Gil reports.

Overall—with Jennie and the thirty-five patients on whom Rappeport and Smith subsequently used anti-Leu 1—the new monoclonal antibody seemed to be effective, but the evidence and the experience, like so much in bone marrow transplantation, are equivocal. Though the general idea is apparently on the right track, neither Rappeport and Smith, nor, as far as Rappeport knows, anyone else, is now using anti-Leu 1. He isn't sure this monoclonal antibody is the best instrument for diminishing GVH, but he started looking elsewhere for a solution mostly because of personnel changes at the pharmaceutical company Rappeport and Smith were using that eliminated the good relationship they had enjoyed with their contacts there.

Since Jennie's transplant, they have tried another monoclonal antibody and considered magnetic beads, a new, similar technology. The search for a solution to GVH, one that won't provoke disease that is as bad or worse, goes on because the need for it is unremitting. Rappeport fears terrible bouts with GVH like Peter Lariviere's, dreads fatal ones like Ricky Stott's.

After Jennie's transplant, as before and during it, Gil Gossom continued to insist that Rappeport tell him how his daughter was doing. Jennie says the reassurances Rappeport gave her were never enough. Her father would wait, jangling his keys, until the doctor told him things were all right. Gil was very angry at Rappeport when he first met him, but also says, "He's a nice guy when you get to know him." He says Rappeport has invited the Gossoms to visit in New Hampshire. "He meant it. I know he did."

For Jennie and Nancy, the going with Rappeport stayed rougher. On a clinic visit after the transplant, Jennie, as usual, waited for hours. "The appointment was always at nine, she'd see him at noon," says Nancy. On this occasion, she suggested that

Jennie "say something to him." "She was feeling lousy," Nancy explains, describing Jennie sitting in the waiting room in her gloves and mask.

When Jennie voiced her complaint, however, Rappeport was furious. "The day that becomes an issue," he yelled, "is the day you find a new doctor. We're not running a bakery here."

Jennie, telling the story, starts to excuse Rappeport, talking about the pressure he's under, the people who die, the atmosphere of fear and need in which he lives. Her mother disagrees. Standing in her living room doorway, her hands on her hips, Nancy shakes her head with assurance. "I don't think it has anything to do with doctoring," she says. "It's just the way he is." But realistic woman of experience that she is, she's willing to dismiss, even forgive, his behavior. "I'm that way myself, sometimes," she says.

Nevertheless, at the time, Jennie returned to the waiting room in tears, and her father thought she'd relapsed. "I don't want it to be a bakery line either," she says, "but you want to know they care." Rappeport had terrified her with his threat. In her condition, where would she find another doctor? Other doctors, and nurses, in the clinic reassured her: of course she wouldn't have to find another doctor. But Jennie, years later, happy and comfortable with her life, cringes into a corner of her living room couch. She is petite, short and slim with small hands and feet. Her movements are both light and controlled—delicate. "You're at their mercy," Jennie says, her enactment of vulnerability refreshing the familiar phrase.

"When he left for New Haven," Gil says, "we were scared."

"I felt abandoned," Jennie says. "You get this bond, you know? I felt that closeness with him. Every time I'd see him after the transplant, he'd say, 'Okay, how many days are we now?' We'd count together. Stuff like that." Again, she acknowledges the difficulty she's had with his personality. "But I admire him so. He's a very smart doctor. And in the long run, I kept saying, Look what he's done for me. How could I ever forget what he's done for me? He's gotten me this far in my life. If I had been anyplace else, or with some other doctor, maybe I wouldn't be so lucky."

SIX

Experimentation

*D*aniel Folsom's bone marrow transplant was an experiment. Scientifically, it was well considered: research gains were commensurate with expectations. Medically, it was justified: Daniel was sure to die without it, almost certainly within the year. It was longed for. Daniel's mother, Reba, is an intelligent woman, and by 1982, the year of the transplant, she was knowledgeable about his disease and bent on preserving her child's life. And yet, in personal terms, it failed, perhaps because of administrative realities, perhaps because of the shortcomings of people who had, or should have had, the power to help the Folsom family.

Wilford Daniel Folsom—called Daniel by his relatives and Danny by his doctors—was Reba and Ezra Folsom's second child, born on March 1, 1974, into the rural north Florida community where both his parents had always lived. Ezra and Reba grew up on adjoining farms. At the time of Daniel's birth, throughout his illness, and for a couple of years after it, the Folsoms ran a land-clearing business and, on their own farm, raised chickens, some cows, and a variety of crops: hay, watermelons, "anything that would bring in income," Reba says.

The Folsoms' feeling for their home and place, like Jennie Gossom's for hers, is firm and deep. The Folsoms' Florida is distinctively Southern: Spanish moss hangs from oak trees, pines are abundant, and palm trees, planted for decoration, live outdoors. The local river is the Suwanee. Towns are small, often with populations of under a thousand people, and names repeat themselves: Buchanan, Reba's maiden name, is also Ezra's first name. People try to keep their land in the family and rarely sell to outsiders.

Churches—all Protestant—are important. Reba is a Southern Baptist, a regular churchgoer and a strong believer, anticipating reunion in heaven with the people she loves. "I just hope all my family gets there."

Reba wears button earrings that match her clothes—red one day, black another—has clear, smooth skin and thick shortish hair. She is carefully groomed and made up, with thin arched eyebrows and bright lipstick. She smokes, but her small, perfectly even teeth are white. She is short, heavy, and muscular.

Reba was twenty when Daniel was born; her husband was in his early thirties. Their elder son, Ezra, Jr., was then three. He was a healthy little boy and had been a normal baby. But Daniel, right from the start, got infection after infection. In December 1974, when Daniel was nine months old, "He developed another ear infection," Reba says. "It was just one right after another, but with this one he had a real high fever."

Reba took him to the emergency room of the local, very small hospital, where the doctor—a general practitioner she had known for years—checked the baby. "He said that his spleen and his liver was very hard. And 'I need you back in the office first thing in the morning.'

"So we carried him back the next morning. The doctor didn't say anything. And it scared me." The doctor drew blood. "He gave him something for the infection, and he started calling a hematologist. He found one at Shands hospital in Gainesville," sixty-five miles away. The area in which the Folsoms live is too sparsely populated to support medical specialists. "I said, 'What are we looking for? What is going on?' " Reba's voice has a musical drawl, but her enunciation is precise. "He said, 'I think he has leukemia.' "

It was worse than that. "We went on down," Reba says of the family's first visit to the hospital in Gainesville, "and they kept doing tests and did a bone marrow. And it took them three days to find out he had Gaucher's disease. And then they took us down to a genetics counselor, that could tell us about it. That there was an enzyme missing in his body and that it was hereditary. And I said, 'Well, I don't know anything about this. How would he get it?' And they said, 'Probably both of you are carriers.' "

Because of the missing enzyme, Daniel's body did not properly rid itself of fats—lipids—in the cells. "So they were storing in his liver. And in his spleen. And he had this large stomach. It was bigger than the rest of him. It made the rest of him look real small. So I asked what they could do about it. And they said there was nothing they could do."

Gaucher's disease is a common genetic disorder that seriously harms a small percentage of the people it affects. Some of these are beyond help. In the most serious of the three types of Gaucher's disease, death by the age of two or three is inevitable. Dr. Edward Ginns, the pediatric neurologist at the National Institutes of Health who participated in Daniel's care, uses the medical term *fulminant* in describing the course of this type—type 2. The symptoms are so severe, manifest themselves so early, and move so quickly that these patients are not candidates for bone marrow transplantation; their brains would be radically and hopelessly damaged before a cure could be effected.

Most people with Gaucher's disease, however, have type 1, which is defined by the *lack* of neurological symptoms such as "pinched nerves and spinal cord problems because of bone infringement," Ginns says. They may have other physical problems, including serious ones, but many people with type 1 Gaucher's disease have no disturbing symptoms, and the majority have a normal life span.

Daniel had type 3 Gaucher's disease, meaning that he did not suffer the serious neurological involvement of type 2, but, Ginns says, had "an abnormal movement of his eyes, a lack of ability to move his eyes, which can be very subtle, and a diffusely slow—mildly slow—EEG." (An electroencephalogram is a test used to determine brain wave activity. Normal EEG measurements correlate with neurological well-being.) "And because of that, he had to be changed from a type 1 to a type 3, but his intelligence was normal, and in this group of children we don't see, at the present time, any other neurologic dysfunction."[1]

Daniel also suffered, to an intense—life-threatening—degree, the disorder's other manifestations. Ginns lists these as "low plate-

lets, anemia, low white counts, large liver, large spleen, bone infections, bone collapse, and pinched nerves, or spinal cord problems
because of bone infringement." He points out, however, that the
variable intensity of Gaucher's makes it a poor candidate for prenatal screening done with an eye to aborting an affected fetus. After
all, he says, most people with Gaucher's disease "would resent not
being here." In fact, he goes on, if one carrier has the mutation for
the severe type and the other for the milder, "the milder seems to
protect" so that afflicted offspring get the less intense form of the
disorder. He contrasts Gaucher's with Tay-Sachs, a rarer disease
that afflicts a similar group of people but is a more reasonable
candidate for such testing—and has a higher profile—because it is
"uniformly lethal."

Gaucher's disease, like Tay-Sachs, occurs most frequently in
Ashkenazi Jews—Jews of German and Eastern European ancestry—and is the most common genetic disease in that ethnic group.
Ginns says one in every twelve or thirteen Ashkenazi Jews is a
carrier. It is not, however, restricted to that group. Rappeport says
that when he first met the Folsoms, they said, "Before you ask,
we're not Jewish. Until we got involved with doctors, we never
even met a Jew."

Gaucher's is an autosomal recessive disease. *Autosomal* means
that the mutation is not on one of the sex-determining chromosomes, X or Y (unlike, for instance, Wiskott-Aldrich syndrome,
which is X-linked). Instead, it is on one of the chromosomes, numbered 1 through 22, each of which is a different size from the
others, with varying numbers and sizes of genes. The gene that is
affected in Gaucher's disease is on chromosome 1, the largest chromosome. *Recessive* means that both parents must carry the defective
gene in order for a child to be afflicted; such a child must inherit
two abnormal chromosomes, one from each parent, each with an
allele (alternative form of a gene) defective at the same locus.

By contrast, in a dominant autosomal disease, inheriting only
one defective allele will cause the problem; the other chromosome
of any given pair will not compensate. Carriers of dominant autosomal diseases, therefore, are always afflicted themselves, and each
of their children—assuming the other parent is normal—has a 50
percent chance of inheriting it. There are no examples of autosomal
dominant diseases in this book. All the people with genetic disease
that I describe and discuss either have autosomal recessive disease,
such as Daniel Folsom with Gaucher's, and the baby with osteo-

petrosis whose donor's marrow was T-cell-depleted, or have sex-linked disease, such as the Wiskott-Aldrich syndrome from which Brian Murphy and Patrick Hough suffered. Rappeport describes a third pattern of inherited disease: codominant, where the manifestations of illness are the result of defects on two different chromosomes, a dynamic whereby "you have two traits that result in a conglomerate disease."

In an autosomal recessive disease, a child of two carriers has a 50 percent chance of being a carrier also, but only a 25 percent chance of actually having the disorder. Reba and Ezra, Daniel's parents, in addition to having one abnormal chromosome, each have a normal chromosome 1 that produces—through the activity of the glucocerebrosidase gene—the enzyme glucocerebrosidase, the function of which is to break down glucocerebroside, in amounts adequate to their needs. In the glucocerebrosidase gene, a number of variations have been shown to cause Gaucher's disease. Ezra's and Reba's abnormal chromosomes, however, are abnormal in the same way, determined by a disarrangement of DNA's famous four "building blocks," identified by the letters A, G, C, and T.

"In Danny's case," says Ginns, "it was a single base change—where there should have been a T there was a C. I think I can show you." He is sitting in a conference room in a huge building on NIH's enormous "campus," showing me slides and diagrams, and referring to Daniel's chart and his own memory of treatment that took place nearly a decade earlier. He clicks the slide projector. "Here it is. His mutation was just below the center of the chromosome"—what Brian Smith describes as "the pinch," the indentation between the arms of a chromosome—"this is where glucocerebrosidase is genetically coded for. And the defect is here, in both his mother's chromosome and his father's chromosome. Each had the defect Danny had, each had the mutation—here—that didn't allow normal glucocerebrosidase to be made within the cells."[2] (The names for enzymes are usually the same as for the substance upon which they act, with the suffix -*ase* added: glucocerebrosid*ase* action is on glucocerebroside.)

For normal function, the human body requires the action of hundreds of thousands of enzymes, proteins that break down other substances, allowing their digestion and elimination. In Gaucher's disease, the absence of just one—the enzyme glucocerebrosidase—results in lipid lying undissolved within cells, in a component outside the nucleus called the lysosome. Gaucher's is therefore classified as a "lysosomal storage disease," in which macrophages, those white cells (also known as histiocytes) whose function is to scavenge for debris, become filled with waste instead of ridding the body of it. The transformed macrophages are known as "Gaucher's cells." Pictures of them, in slides and textbooks, show strands of glucocerebroside wound, like thread or yarn, around and around the nucleus, or in some cases the nuclei. Hematologists describe the huge cells as swollen, or pregnant, or—most aptly—constipated.

Gaucher's cells spared Daniel Folsom's brain. "I think everyone would say he was intellectually very bright," Ginns says. "He was special," Reba says. "And not just because he was mine." "Everyone was always impressed," says Ginns. "There was no neurologic impairment," say Ginns and Rappeport, identically but separately. "His intelligence was perfectly normal." The doctors make this point because it would not have been ethical to transplant Daniel if there had been the severe neurological impairment of type 2 disease. Gaucher's cells, however, invaded his spleen, his liver, his bones, his lungs, and his bone marrow.

After Daniel was diagnosed in Gainesville, the Folsoms took him home. "It was almost Christmas," Reba says. "And I was raised in a way that—you don't question. I was very religious, I was born and raised in a Christian home. And I felt very selfish when I was standing at the sink that night when I came home, and I was washing dishes, and it finally hit me. And I just started screaming, Why, why, did it have to happen? To me? And I felt very guilty about doing that."

Until Daniel was diagnosed, neither of his parents had ever heard of Gaucher's disease, and they do not know now of any cases of it on either side of the family, although "my husband's grandfather died at a very young age," Reba says. "And he looked like Daniel did—so I was told. He had the large stomach. He died of mysterious reasons. Back then they said everybody died of pneumonia, because they didn't have anything to treat those things. But it was a very mysterious death. And that was the only thing we thought might—would make a connection." Reba says "there was a lot of blaming" on both sides of the family. " 'Oh, I know where that came from,' it came from your mother's side, or it came from some of your background, you know. It was bad. And there were a lot of hurt feelings—there were a lot of people that were all upset, that something was wrong with him. And I didn't need that. And naturally Daniel didn't need to hear that.

"We went on, he kept having the ear infections, and he kept going back to have his blood checked, and they kept telling us there was nothing they could do about it." Reba means by this that doctors did not offer a cure. Throughout his illness, they did treat him: with antibiotics and blood transfusions, with surgery and with casts. Because of his low platelet count, his spleen was removed when he was three. At about the same time, his bones started breaking. "One day—I was on a woman's softball team, and he was sitting in the dugout with me, and he stepped down off the bench and started limping. And I said, 'Are you okay?' And he said, 'My hip hurts.' And I said, 'Well, I better take you to the doctor, I guess.' So we waited overnight, and the next day I carried him, and they found out that he had fractured his hip. He didn't fall or anything, he just stepped down. They never mentioned to me that it would deteriorate the bones."

As Reba tells her story, it is this recurring point—the lack of information or explanation given her—that angers her, even more than the cruelty of fate. "They didn't *tell* me that," she says at various junctures. Whether or not the people in question knew the relevant facts is immaterial to her. In another context, telling me about an ancestor who suffered from what is now presumed to have been epilepsy, Reba criticized the ill-treatment the long-dead woman endured. "There's no excuse for ignorance," she said, "with all there is to read. Ignorance is just stupid," but her real grievance with other people is not their lack of knowledge. It is their unwillingness or incapacity to confront, with her, the issues and problems that trouble her. All the betrayals Reba perceives derive from a lack of communication, a failure of other people to involve themselves with her worry and sorrow.

My mother once said that she could bear Roberta's illness "because I'm in on everything." At the very end, an hour or two before my sister fell into a coma, she looked up, frightened, at my mother. Roberta had spent six years struggling for her life. Rappeport later told me, paying a high compliment, that she and Reba were unique, in his experience, for the degree of their purposeful tenacity. When she died, Roberta was fifty-one, and by then her wisdom was great and her patience limitless, but the person in the reclining chair was the child, the adolescent I remembered from our shared youth. Her body was swollen in the middle from steroids and wasted at the extremities from illness, but it communicated a need that evoked the teenaged Roberta, a girl eager—almost wild—to give and receive affection and reassurance, and so re-minded me of my own body, of life. I cannot say what effect it had on my mother, who had grieved before, and now knew that she would grieve forever, but she bent over her child, with her shaking hand touched Roberta's face and hair, and said, responding to the words that had not been spoken, "You won't even know. You won't even know it's happening." And Roberta was comforted.

Reba, speaking of her years of intimacy with Daniel's illness, says she never kept anything from him. "He had become—he was a part of *me*. He needed me. And I needed him at that point." And so she informed him, as she wanted to be informed herself, and she stayed with him. "I never left him, in all those years. He was handicapped, he was sick, and he needed me. If he was afraid—of a procedure or something—I'd say, 'No big deal. It's going to hurt. But I'll be there with you.' And he got comfort from that. He knew that I would never leave his bed."

At home, Reba managed Daniel's care, nursing him through the crises that became more and more frequent. His bones broke both because of infection that was a result of his Gaucher's-compromised bone marrow and because Gaucher's cells had dimin-ished the ability of the bones' cells—the osteoclasts and osteoblasts—to break down and repair themselves properly. "They put him in a cast," Reba says, describing treatment for Daniel's first known fracture, "a body cast, from just above his belly button down. And his legs. And said that hopefully it would heal. But it didn't. He stayed in a body cast, he couldn't sit up or anything. I set up a hospital bed in the living room, where he could watch TV and everything."

After six weeks the doctors took the cast off, found Daniel's hip still not healed, put a pin in it, and put the body cast on for another six weeks. "Then we got him back on his feet again, and he was using a hand walker." He was not yet four. "He wouldn't be falling or anything, and every time you turned around it seemed like he had a fracture in his leg. Or he had a fracture in his finger. And then he was having the vertebraes in his back do the same thing. They would just fracture and give way, there was no fall or anything that caused them. We got him back on his feet again, though, after that other pin was put in. They wanted to go ahead and get another pin and put it in his other hip, to try to support it," in order to prevent further damage, "but in the X rays you could see a hairline fracture every time there was a break." And about the same time, "You could notice a change in his breathing." Gaucher's cells had invaded his lungs.

Nevertheless, Reba says, "We went along real well there for about a year. Didn't have too many problems." And so, when Reba's parents and youngest sister decided to travel to Omaha to visit another sister then living there—Reba is one of seven children—she decided to go, taking along young Ezra and four-and-a-half-year-old Daniel, eager for the trip. Ezra, Sr., stayed home. "We had a big farm," Reba says, "and you have to stay with it if you're going to make the crop."

The family traveled in two cars. "We were going to have plenty of room; we carried all the necessary things to make Daniel's ride comfortable. My mother had this fear of planes, so we wouldn't fly. Daniel and Ezra and I and my mother and my dad and my baby sister left one morning about five o'clock. And when we got to Mississippi, Daniel started showing signs of fatigue." Reba's father wasn't feeling well either; something they'd eaten at a fast-food restaurant seemed to have made both Daniel and his grandfather sick. "And by the time we got to Omaha, to my sister's house, Daniel had a real high fever." Reba called Daniel's doctors in Florida, who told her to take him to Children's Hospital in Omaha.

They went instead to the Methodist Hospital, where in the past Reba's sister had taken her family. Daniel was diagnosed as having yet another ear infection, given an antibiotic, and sent home again. "We carried him home, back to my sister's, and that night his fever went so high we couldn't get it down. We had him in the tub, washing him down, cooling him off. The next morning, he was lethargic. He didn't recognize anybody. It scared me to death. And we carried him back to the emergency room at Methodist Hospital, and they made— They sent us over to Children's." There, they put him into intensive care.

"The doctor said, 'I don't think Daniel's going to make it.' Well, I wasn't ready for anything like that. I said, 'No, he's not going to die.' And he said, 'We don't know what's wrong with him. Until we get some of these cultures back.' And it took them almost three days. I didn't leave him. I *never* left him, always stayed with him. And they told us that he had salmonella food poisoning." Presumably from the fast-food meal, from which Reba's father easily recovered. "That's the only link I can find," says Reba. "They thought he had spinal meningitis because of all the symptoms. After they found out it was salmonella, then they knew what to give him, and he started coming out of it. When he looked at me and said, 'I'm fine,' I couldn't help but scream. Everybody thought I was crazy in intensive care, but I really thought I was going to lose him, because they didn't have any hope for him.

"He overcame that, and he got herpes, and his mouth would break out in real bad sores. His mouth was so sore he could hardly eat. He was so hungry; he'd been without food for so many days, and he would eat. I would feed him, and the sores would bust and they would bleed. And I'd clean him up, and he'd say, 'I'm still hungry,' so I'd keep feeding him. We stayed out there—I guess four weeks, in the hospital. Four weeks."

With the Omaha hospitalization, the Folsoms incurred the first of their enormous medical debts. They carried no medical insurance. Reba says this is because Ezra did not think it necessary. "He always felt that if you had a life insurance policy—or two—that you could borrow from the insurance policies and pay the hospital bills. Well, that was fine when we didn't have any medical problems. But after Daniel was born, it was too late; we could not get medical insurance on him."

In Florida, the state paid nearly all Daniel's expenses. He was treated out of state as well: in Omaha, in Atlanta, in Maryland at the National Institutes of Health, and—for the transplant—in Boston. At the NIH, treatment was free, as it always is there, but in Atlanta and Omaha, the Folsoms had to pay for all Daniel's care.

Daniel went from the Omaha Hospital to the one in Gainesville. Reba wanted him back in Florida, where he was soon to start kindergarten, and so the doctors in Nebraska "arranged for Shands," the hospital in Gainesville, "to take him back so we could get closer to home, and that was in August. And we brought him back and carried him straight to Shands," where he stayed for another four weeks. "It was time for school to start, and he couldn't start to school." The teacher sent books, and Reba taught him. "We started learning—because he already knew some of his ABC's and stuff, and he could write his name and all. We started working on it, so when he got out of the hospital, he says, 'Well, I'm ready to go to school.' But by this time—through the salmonella, the stress, Gaucher's, everything—he couldn't walk. So I told my father, 'I want you to go down to the medical supply place and get me a wheelchair where he can go to school.' Because he was looking forward to it so much. I went to school with him for six weeks, every day. We lived ten, twelve miles from school. I drove him to school, I stayed with him all day, to push him around, help him to go to the bathroom—because he couldn't stand up very well—and just to be there when he needed to be moved, because I didn't want anything to break."

Then, "I went to the school board and told them that, by law, they had to put an aide there for him. And they did." Reba knew her rights because she had called members of Congress. "I made a few calls to congressmen, and they were very helpful, the congressmen was. I called and asked them, I told them, 'I've got this son that is physically handicapped. Mentally he is not. Physically he is. And I have to go to school with him for him to be able to go.' They said, 'Well, why don't we just put him homebound?' I said, 'No, I don't want him different from the other kids.' " And, says Reba, he wasn't. "The kids accepted him and played with him, would take him out of the wheelchair and sit him on the floor. The kids in the class would all sit down on the floor and play with him wherever he was, because they knew he couldn't get up and play with them."

Young Ezra helped, too. At this time, he was in the third grade. Reba took him to school also, and she saw to it that he played Little League. "I wanted Ezra to be as much like the other kids as possible. I didn't want to make him feel that he had to give things up just because Daniel was disabled." But "We had a big farm, and I had chores to do. I couldn't leave Daniel in the house by himself, so I'd put him on the floor with his toys, and Ezra would get down and play with him, because Ezra was big enough so he could pick him up and move him if he needed to, or in case of a fire or something he could move him out. Or if something happened he would be there with him. And I would go out and do my chores until five, six o'clock in the evening and then I'd come in and fix dinner. But Ezra would give up a lot of things to take care of Daniel."

One afternoon when she was in the house and Ezra was outside playing with his brother, a rattlesnake came up beside the two children. Ezra picked Daniel up and brought him into the house, and Reba picked up a shotgun and fired but failed to kill the snake. Ezra took the gun from her hands, finished off the rattler, and then carried his brother outside again. At this time, Ezra was not yet ten years old.

When Ezra was eighteen, and in the army, he wrote to me

about his family and their experience with Daniel's illness. His first letter is dated "5 Jan 90." He was in basic training.

> Daniel was a very special person to me. I really loved him a lot. I still think of him often. When we learned of the possibility of a transplant I wanted to be the donor from the beginning. Maybe I wanted to be the hero that saved his life. Then again I sometimes wonder if I was just jealous of all the attention he got. Maybe I wanted to be the donor where I could have some of the spotlight. But you know how kids think.
>
> Deep down I don't think that I was jealous. I was only 10 at the time of the actual transplant. I do not really know what I was thinking. I made the donation out of love. It's the only thing I could do for him. I wasn't pressured into anything but I was informed that I was his only hope.
>
> I am so glad that you are undertaking the job of writing this book. So many people do not understand the heartaches, the joys and everything involved with this miraculous piece of medical science!
>
> I know that this is an unorganized letter but I hope you can make some sense out of it. It's hard to think in the Army at times and this is one of them times.
>
> Many times I felt neglected by my Mom. I knew that she was doing something important but it seemed at the time that I had important needs. I guess that is why we are so close now. We are still making up for lost time.
>
> My father was never very emotional during the whole ordeal. I guess he was trying to show that real men don't cry. He was wrong. He loved all of us, but he had a hard time of showing it. But I understand him now. Though he never really showed it I know that he was hurting inside.

"There's something in Ezra that you don't see in an eighteen-year-old boy, normally," Reba says. "The respect and concern for others."

"I always— I wouldn't settle for less than the best," Reba says. She is talking about finding care for Daniel. "Anytime we went anywhere, I asked questions. Constantly. 'What are you doing to him?' or, 'What are you planning on doing to him?' Or, 'What have you found out?' " In Florida, the doctor in charge "didn't want to tell me these things. Like, 'You wouldn't understand.' Well, hell, I may not understand, but if you'll sit there long enough you can *make* me understand. Now, he was a good doctor. We had a lot of clashes in personality. They were dealing with a country hick, and here I am with all these doctors, you know, who are supposed to know everything. Anyway, they found out that I wasn't so stupid after all.

"When we got back from Omaha, and Daniel was still in Shands, there was a resident on the case. He only came in for just a few times. He said, 'They're researching Gaucher's disease somewhere. And I intend to find it.' He told me that there was a place in England, and then he found out that there was NIH. And he said, 'I'm going to do what I can to get you there.' " Reba thinks this young man's name was Dr. Norman, but she is not sure. She would like to remember, because she wants to give him credit for what he did. Other doctors were mentioned "in the medical journals and all, about being involved. But he wasn't. That's what kills me. Because he was the one that did all the research to find the place to go. He was never recognized, and he was the turning point for me, I felt. He was the hope that I had. Because nobody else had given me any hope.

"He told me, 'We've gotten in touch with the genetics people at the National Institutes of Health in Bethesda, Maryland.'

"I said, 'And?'

" 'Well, they are researching the disease, and they want to see Daniel.' "

Ed Ginns first saw Daniel Folsom in September 1980. Ginns, who had come to work in John Barranger's laboratory, had then been at the NIH for only three months. Before that, he had earned a Ph.D. in physical chemistry, served in the Public Health Service for three years, graduated from medical school, and completed a residency in neurology. He came to the NIH specifically to work on Gaucher's disease, and Daniel was one of the first patients with the disorder he saw. "I hadn't seen many Gaucher's patients at this point, but he looked terrible," Ginns said.[3]

"At this point," says Reba, "you could look at Daniel and you'd just think something was wrong with his legs—that he couldn't walk—because he was in a wheelchair. You wouldn't think that all these things were wrong inside." The main problems at this time, and until the transplant, were the infections and fractures with which the Folsoms were already familiar ("including compression fractures of all vertebrae," says the scientific paper written after the transplant)[4] and cirrhosis of the liver—a result of Gaucher's cells infiltrating that organ—and, secondary to that, hemor-rhaging of the esophageal varices.

"Some very small percentage of Gaucher patients," Ginns explains, "including Danny, actually go through the stages similar to alcoholic, cirrhotic livers, where the liver just can't keep up with whatever's toxic. Eventually there's liver dysfunction and scarring, and then the blood can't go through the liver and goes through collateral vessels. One of those is esophageal, and that leads to esophageal varices." Rappeport describes esophageal varices as "hemorrhoids of the esophagus," the passage from the pharynx to the stomach. "As the pressure gets higher there," says Ginns, "the blood is shunted off to the varices into blood vessels that get bigger and bigger to accommodate the flow." The varices erode—through eating and other normal functions—"and that's where Danny was bleeding."

Daniel's symptoms had not yet made the Folsoms aware of this danger, but they would recognize it soon, and then they would have to start elaborate stopgap measures to prevent catastrophic bleeding from the esophageal varices, a critical part of Daniel's treatment before and beyond the transplant. At the time of the Folsoms' first visits to the NIH, however, Ginns and Barranger and their colleagues offered information and suggested some measures to increase Daniel's comfort—for instance, Ginns says, he was fitted with lightweight braces so that he could get around better, as he was determined to do.

"I came to the realization," says Reba, "that I'm not going to have him that long. That he is going to die."

"A regular hospital," says Ginns, "sees these patients and says, 'Oh, God, what do we do, this patient is at death's door.' But our threshold is much higher." His group wanted to find out more about Gaucher's disease. "All the patients [at the NIH] need to be seen on a protocol, meaning a particular group is interested in research on what the patient has. And many of these patients represent the only way we get samples and are able to study the disease."

"They told me," says Reba, speaking of Ginns and Barranger, "anytime something happened to Daniel, to let them know. If I didn't mind. So I did. I had a lot of confidence in these two guys. They had—maybe you'd call it a good bedside manner? Or maybe they truly cared. I don't really think it was all a show. And also, it would help them with the research, too. I realize that. Lots of times

I think we got caught up in the research. And lots of times I felt like we were being used. Because I thought they knew more than they were telling me."

Again, ignorance is, for Reba, an almost unbearably frustrating issue. She says that at the NIH she found out Daniel was likely to live only until his teens, and that until then she didn't know that "he had progressed this much, and that all these things could happen to him. And I was angry then. I can't believe that a teaching hospital like Shands, with all these people, all these doctors there, and these so-called specialists, did not know all these problems that goes along with the Gaucher's disease. I can't believe that. I just felt like they didn't want to bother to tell me, or maybe they didn't think that I would understand. I don't know. That's when the anger started building at Shands."

Other events at Shands added to Reba's travail and to her dislike of the people there. One time, Daniel fell out of bed and broke his leg, and when the Folsoms brought him to the emergency room, they were cross-examined about child abuse, despite Reba's pleas to get the orthopedist familiar with her child's case and to pull the chart that would explain Daniel's difficulty to her questioners. And there was the infuriating instance when a doctor told Reba she was "too attached" to her child. "Do you have children?" Reba asked. "Yes," said the doctor, "I have two children." "Do you love 'em?" "And we really got off on a bad note when I asked her that. She says, 'Yeah, but I don't think I'd be attached.' I said, 'Wait a minute. Have you ever had a sick child? You ever had a problem like this?' 'Well, no, I can't say I have.' I said, 'You can't understand what I'm feeling.' She and I didn't get along at all. And I asked them to just remove her from the case.

"Because anybody unfeeling like that, not letting *me* express *my* feelings, and try to understand what-all's going on—I don't need that kind of person around me.

"Any negative attitudes at that point in my life, I didn't want them around me. While Daniel was going through all these years of pain, it would make me physically sick, and it still does, to this day, to hear someone say, 'Oh, my back hurts.' I don't even ask anybody, 'How're you doing?' anymore. Because, certain ones, everything in the world is wrong with them. And I just think, You don't know, you just can't begin to know the pain I saw. You can't begin to know what I've seen in all these hospitals I've been in.

"It was like you take care of one problem, okay, everything looks good, you know? Everything's not so bad after all. You take care of another problem. Well, he's getting better, maybe they don't know what they're talking about. This is what I was going through until I got to NIH and found out that I didn't know anything. I did not know anything about Gaucher's disease, because those people at Gainesville didn't tell me nothing. And that pissed me off in a hurry. That's when I started losing confidence in the people at Shands. It was like, Why are you doing this to me? All I want to know is some answers. You know, Can you do anything? Or, What's going to happen to him? What do I need to expect, so I won't be shocked? But there was a lot of things that a lot of them didn't tell me—even NIH didn't tell me—that could possibly happen to him."

Ed Ginns says, "To people who don't see a lot of Gaucher cells, the cell can look like a B lymphocyte, and children are misdiagnosed as having leukemia. Many children, when they get to the NIH, have already had a bone marrow biopsy to 'stage' their disease, and it's a surprise when the pathology report comes back and says they don't have leukemia, they have Gaucher's disease. Sometimes that good news—the majority are better off with Gaucher—but sometimes it's bad."[5]

At the NIH, in the beginning, Reba says, "They told me they didn't have anything to offer Daniel at the time. They had been trying enzyme replacement with some of the adult patients and had not seen any remarkable improvement. And maybe when something came up, they would consider Daniel. So I said, 'You mean, I'm going to go back home, and I'm just going to wait?' And they said, 'And take care of the immediate problems. Whatever comes up.'

"We come back from the NIH. I don't even remember what month it was." It would have been the late fall or early winter of 1980. "One night, we were at some kind of reunion or function of some kind, and Daniel had to throw up. And I took him outside, and he threw up blood. And I didn't know what was happening—this is one of the things they didn't tell me to expect. We immediately left and went home. I don't know why we went home. I don't know why we didn't just get in the car and go to the hospital with him. But it wasn't a lot of blood, and my husband says, 'Well, he probably got a cold, or something he ate.' 'Cause the blood, it wasn't fresh blood, it looked like old blood. And he had drunk a Coke, and my husband seemed to think that that might have been what it was. Anyway, we went home and Daniel told me, 'I have to go to the bathroom.' And when he did, we found out he had the tarry stools. I'd never seen that before. And it just has an awful smell. And I said, 'Something is terribly wrong.' So before we could get dressed to go to the hospital, I had laid Daniel back on the bed, after he went to the bathroom, and all of a sudden he says, 'I gotta throw up.' And when he did, it was just all this fresh blood, just everywhere. 'Oh, God,' I said. I was hysterical. I said, 'Get your clothes on.' We didn't even take time to call an ambulance. Where we lived up there it would have taken forever to get an ambulance. We didn't have one in our county. We would've had to wait for one to come from another county to get there to get him. So we just jumped in the car and left. And we headed for Gainesville. We got stopped for speeding, and we told him what was going on, and they went on ahead and called Shands. And we got there, and all I wanted to do was get the hematologists, because, I said, they're the ones that deal with Daniel, because he's bleeding and I didn't know how to go about stopping the bleeding.

"They started—they put him in intermediate care at Shands, in the children's wing, and they put a tube down. I was scared to death. I didn't know what was going on, and they still couldn't— they wouldn't— 'Right now, we've got to deal with Daniel, we'll talk to you later.' And I understood that, but I was so afraid—I didn't know what was going on. I—didn't—know—what—to—expect."

As doctors in Massachusetts had done when Peter Lariviere's ulcer started bleeding, doctors at Shands were practicing lavage on Daniel, forcing a cold solution down into his stomach—he was conscious throughout the procedure—and then bringing it back out. They stopped the bleeding that night and told Reba that she could take Daniel home in the morning.

"But that morning it just started all over again. And they started this lavage again, trying to stop the bleeding. They got it stopped again. They put us in a regular room. And at this point, they had no earthly idea what to do with him."

"While they were working on Daniel," Reba says, "I called Dr. Barranger and Ginns at NIH, and said, 'Hey, Daniel started bleeding.' I gave them the whole story about the tarry stools and what the Shands doctors were doing." Ginns and Barranger suggested sclerosing Daniel's esophageal varices. There was a doctor in Atlanta—a pediatric gastroenterologist named Daniel Caplan—whom they recommended to do the procedure. "Dr. Ginns explained it to me. They would inject a solution into the varices, and it would close them off, it would seal off the veins that were enlarged. Just like you would, I guess, in a varicose vein in your leg."

Rappeport, who was not yet involved in Daniel's care—he and the Folsoms did not meet, or even hear of each other, until shortly before the transplant—is dubious about the sclerosing procedure. He says it was not well studied at the time it was carried out on Daniel and that it carries a risk of infection. He thinks transfusion may have been a wiser course, but sclerosing was a regular part of Daniel's life before Rappeport was, and doctors at the NIH had faith in the procedure and in Dr. Caplan throughout.

Ginns and Barranger contacted Caplan, and he agreed to treat Daniel. "When it came time for us to figure out how we were going to get him to Atlanta," Reba says, "Shands would not release him to go by ambulance. That was a long ways. It's a six-hour drive. Or any other way, but by flying him." The Folsoms chartered a plane. "We made the arrangements, got them to help us to make the arrangements to have emergency medical set up on the plane, and to fly him there with a med tech. Daniel and I flew up, and his father drove up with Ezra.

"I met Dr. Caplan, and he told me the procedure, how they would go in and seal off these veins. And stop it from happening again. But with cirrhosis of the liver, it always comes back. If one vein is sealed off, another one will develop. He was very good at explaining this to me. And he said, 'If you don't get him to a hospital, he's always going to bleed—he'll bleed to death if you don't get him there.' And that was always my fear. I lived sixty-five miles from Gainesville, and was I going to get him there each time? Because it happened, over and over and over again."

That first time, "They carried him in and sclerosed him. And he was fine, and he was in a good mood. By this time, though, his potassium was down, and he started acting real lethargic, so they had to build that back up. He'd lost a lot of blood; they had to replace his blood. He received a lot of blood, all those years." And everything—the doctors' fees, the drugs, the hospital costs, the price of chartering a plane—was at the Folsoms' expense because, again, they were uninsured and out of the state of Florida. "Anyway, we got it done, and Dr. Caplan told me that it was possible that it would happen again. And it did. It wasn't very long that it happened again. We went back through the same procedure again. We went back to Shands. We went through the whole nine yards of chartering a plane. Four or five times, before we ever went to Boston." All this was happening before the curative possibility—the transplant—was proposed.

Meanwhile, the Folsoms' relationship with the NIH continued. "We'd made numerous trips back and forth to the NIH, whenever they needed to do more skin tests, or needed some more blood, or maybe a liver test, or something, to check his progression." And Daniel's life went on as normally as Reba could make it. He went to school, finishing kindergarten—Reba talks with pride about a graduation ceremony, when Daniel wheeled himself across the floor—and first grade and second. "After the bleeding started—that was terrible. That was a problem for me, to have to stay away from him during the day with that aide at school. But I always made sure that someone was near the phone, and I would give the school my mother's number and my sister's, because they were close by and could be there, or find me. Because if I was outside working, someone would have to find me."

Daniel was now seven years old. His prognosis was terrible. Ginns says, "He really was, if not the severest, one of the most severe the program had seen here. We figured that he'd die in the next year or two, and that he had *no* chance of living for five more years if something wasn't done."[6]

"That was our criteria." For Daniel to have a bone marrow transplant. Since one had never been performed on a person with Gaucher's disease, it was ethically essential that the candidate be someone for whom there was no realistic hope of life without the procedure. Otherwise the risks—both known and unforeseeable—were untenable. Because this little boy was very, very sick, desperately in need of anything that could be done for him, he was an opportunity, a laboratory.

In May of 1981, Daniel was admitted to the NIH for reevaluation and consideration for a bone marrow transplant. At the time, bone marrow transplants were not performed at the hospital there. Ginns remembers that several medical centers were considered and "my recollection is that Boston Children's Hospital by itself had a fantastic reputation—still has a fantastic reputation. And Joel's interest was not just in aplastics and leukemics but had broadened out to genetic disorders." Rappeport's intense attentiveness to individual patients was also a factor.

The terms of the experiment were always clear.

"The reason you can do a transplant," says Ginns, speaking after the fact, "and try to effect a therapy in this disorder, is that even though all the tissues are missing a functional enzyme to some degree, the storage seems to occur almost exclusively in the macrophages, which come from monocytes, which come from the bone marrow."

Barranger says Gaucher's is unique among lysosomal storage diseases in that storage is only in the macrophage.[7]

"A little storage occurs in endothelial cells, which are the cells that line the blood vessels," Ginns says, but virtually all storage is in the macrophage, "the garbage pail, where everything gets dumped. So the theory was that because all the stored lipid seems somehow to get shuttled to the macrophages—in the kidney, in the spleen—then even if the liver, the spleen, the kidney, and the brain are not replaced and still have the genetic defect, replacement of the macrophages would be effective treatment. We don't know yet what happens in the brain." (A scientist, reporting at the American Society of Hematology's 1990 meeting, said that a Swedish child transplanted for Gaucher's disease shortly after Daniel Folsom was, is now showing some signs of neurological deterioration.)[8]

Rappeport cites the background leading to the thesis that a bone marrow transplant would correct Gaucher's disease: Clinical research had shown that in patients who received bone marrow transplants "the liver macrophage called the Kupffer cell would develop the chromosomal markers of the donor. Similarly, the alveolar macrophage in the lung would develop chromosomal material of donor origin. And a little peripherally, what led to the use of this in osteopetrosis was that the osteoclast, which causes reabsorption of the bone, so that there's a constant making and breaking going on, was also of donor origin."

"Nobody knew," Brian Smith says, "if in the storage diseases replacing just the macrophage would take care of the disease."

"Our arrangement with Joel," says Ginns, "was that we could not do anything researchwise that would compromise the transplant course. That the medical treatment came first, and then the research part of it. We hoped it would never come to a decision of one versus the other, but that was the understanding.

"It had never been done," Ginns says. "You can hypothesize with culture in the laboratory however you want, but until you try it, you're not going to know whether it really works or what the risks are."[9]

In June, Reba and Daniel left the NIH and flew to Boston, Reba managing Daniel's fragile body, his wheelchair, and all the new experiences she had to face and assimilate. Before Daniel's sickness, she says, "I never thought I could manage if I had to live more than a mile from my mother." Until Reba started flying in and out of airports with a sick child and anxiety in tow, she had never seen a taxicab, except on television. But she never questioned going. "Dr. Ginns and Barranger suggested that if maybe we do the transplant, replace all the old cells that are there, the body would repair itself. With the bone marrow. Dr. Rappeport didn't know, you know, he couldn't tell them right then. He said, 'I'm going to need to see him.' We carried medical reports with us, from NIH and Shands, and there were more tests at Children's, and X rays and photographs. They took pictures of his torso, of how he looked and all with his clothes off. And to Daniel, that was a degrading feeling. He was a very modest child. He thought people would make fun of him."

The picture reproduced in the scientific report that summarizes the case[10] shows a naked little boy—in the paper his eyes and genitals are covered to convey an anonymity he really didn't have and a privacy he wasn't allowed—with a huge, distended belly, skinny arms and legs, and a round face with full lips, the mouth turned down. Daniel was not able to stand unaided, and a uniformed woman is holding him under the arms; her hand covers nearly a quarter of his torso. "His height and weight," says the report, "were below the third percentile." And the Folsoms are big people.

"They did their tests," Reba says, "and Dr. Rappeport said, 'Well, I'll get back to you. Soon. Give me a chance to go through all these X rays.' So we flew home. We was up there I guess two or three days. We flew home, and we waited. Went through another body cast with his bones. It was always his legs. It seemed he was always in a body cast with his bones breaking. And then went through another couple of bleeds with the esophageal varices. We always had those sclerosed in Atlanta.

"Then we got a phone call. Later in the summer. After dark one night. It was only Daniel and Ezra"—Reba means the younger Ezra—"there at the time. It was Dr. Rappeport, and I'd been just so anxious to hear from him to see what they were going to do, or what they thought they could do. He talked to me—oh, God, I guess he talked to me for an hour on the phone.

"He said, 'We think that maybe the transplant would be a good decision. But it's your decision. Whatever you want to do. I'm going to tell you what could happen, and then you'll have to make the decision.' So he was telling me that Daniel had a fifty-fifty chance of survival with the transplant. He told me all the complications as far as infection's concerned. Everything that goes on in the transplant. He was so informative."

This was the foundation of the trust Reba had in Rappeport, right through to the end. "He told me everything. Daniel's sitting there in his wheelchair listening to me. You know, just waiting to see what I was going to say. Because I looked at him and mouthed that it was Dr. Rappeport.

"And Dr. Rappeport says, 'Well, what do you want to do?' I said, 'I don't know.' Because he told me how risky it was. It was new for Gaucher's disease—they were going into a field they knew very little about, and we didn't know what to expect, only by those who had had the transplants before, for other things. I told him, 'I'll call you back. I have to talk this over with my husband.'

" 'It's your decision,' " Reba quotes Ezra, Sr., as saying, unresolved anger in her voice. "See, it was always like *my* decision. And I hated that. I wanted help with the decision. I didn't want to feel that whatever happened, it's all my fault, you know? I needed help with these decisions, but he says, 'You're with him all the time, you know this—you talk to the doctors a lot.' I said, 'I told you everything the doctors said, and I need some help in this decision.' "

Reba says that Ezra, Sr., not only did not help her make decisions, he also held himself apart from her during the time of fiercest worry about Daniel. She wanted companionship in her terrible responsibility. She remembers a lack of involvement from Ezra when she needed it, and it still gnaws at her. She says that Ezra told her only once, in all the long time of Daniel's illness, that he loved her.

But she also says of her husband's feeling toward Daniel, and toward young Ezra, "He loved him. He loved his children. There was no doubt in my mind that he loved him."

At the time of the transplant, Ezra, Sr., was a big, heavy, brown-haired man. Reba's snapshots show him round-faced, robust, and smiling in his farmer's overalls. Eight year later, he is thin and white-haired, but the impression he makes is, like Reba's, one of force, of internal power, and of high intelligence. He told me, as his son did, that he was glad I was writing this book, that he would be especially interested in reading "what other people have been through."

Ezra Folsom said this as he sat, a cup of coffee on the Formica table in front of him, in a restaurant with Reba and me. He also said, "I'm very emotional, but I don't thrive on letting my emotions out. I just kick my butt and get on out." Ezra, Jr., he said, is the same way. "He had the ability not to think about it too much. He held his grief in, but you could tell he was grieving." And with great firmness he said, "The brothers loved each other." Reba had told me that Ezra, Sr., had longed to be the donor, but to me he was laconic about it: "It wouldn't have created a problem to be a donor."

Long before a bone marrow transplant was proposed for Daniel, Ezra knew about the procedure. This is highly unusual; of the people I interviewed for this book, very few had heard of a bone marrow transplant until they had one or a family member did, and then their knowledge was skimpy and vague, gleaned mostly from publicity about the ones Admiral Zumwalt's son, Elmo Zumwalt, Jr., and Senator Paul Tsongas had received. *No one* I talked to who needed a transplant before the late 1980s had heard of it ahead of time, except Ezra Folsom. He reads a lot, he said—newspapers and magazines—and "I knew the principle, and I knew about the germ-free environment."

Ezra did not believe the bone marrow transplant would help Daniel. "Once his body was deteriorating, you could look into the future and see what was going to happen." He wanted to remember him as a very little child, Ezra said, and he held out his hand a couple of feet above the floor to indicate a toddler's height, "before things got bad."

His recollection was that the doctors in Gainesville said the Folsoms could expect Daniel to live to be thirty or more, but, he says, "They didn't know enough about it, or tell us enough, for us to know what to expect. And then, from the time he fractured his hip, it was tough on us."

Nevertheless, he said, he did want Daniel to have the transplant. Without it, he surely "had no future. His body was devastated; it would have kept on deteriorating without the transplant. And the NIH was interested in the results. The people in Boston were interested." He himself prayed that Daniel would die, long before he did, so that the suffering would end. But, he said, "I wasn't the only one in it." There are people, he says, who have trouble—not necessarily this kind—who can't put it aside and go on. His eyes fill. "My wife believed, up until the day he died, that he would live. And that was worth it. And I don't hold that against her one bit. The love of a mother for a child is wonderful."

The experience with Daniel "hasn't changed our lives," he said. It was true that medical expenses were a problem, and being way from home was, because "it takes you away from business." Missing work was a problem. He said, though, that now "Reba's doing good, I am." When Daniel was sick, "Everybody did everything they could."

Ezra does not have much to say about Rappeport. He believes him to be a good doctor, but he didn't get to know him. "I didn't try. It wasn't a social occasion." But of the people at home, the people he's always known and those he had never met who came forward to help, he said, "You don't realize how many friends you have until you have trouble."

"What he said about 'Reba doing good, I'm doing good.' But it did hurt us,' " Reba said, driving away from the restaurant. "I hated the suffering," she said, speaking of Daniel. "But I couldn't let go of him." There came a time, she said, when she too "used to pray he would die, because of all the suffering."

She is a fast driver; we zoomed past signs that said "No shooting from the road," and the new yellow brick school for eight hundred children, kindergarten through twelfth grade, and mostly past open fields with herds of cattle and stacks of hay. Part of the road was being paved; the asphalt was still completely black, and the smell was strong. Earlier, Reba had tried to describe the appearance and odor of a tarry stool—of Daniel's bowel movements, permeated with old blood. "That's it," she said as we drove along, "that's what it looked like, and that's what it smelled like." Although, then again, it didn't really smell like tar. It was a stronger odor than that, and more foul. "Hell," said Reba, "I don't know what I wanted. I wanted what was best."

"So Daniel is just sitting there all along, listening to us," Reba says, speaking of the night of Rappeport's call, when she and Ezra talked about the prospect of a transplant. "Back and forth about what to do, and Daniel looks at me and he says, 'I want to know. What did Dr. Rappeport say?' And I told him about the infection he could get, that it could be fatal. I told him about the possibility of it not working. I told him of his chances of survival if he didn't take this chance. What I was feeling, though, all I could think about was Daniel dying. If this was going to be something that could kill him, would he live longer without it?

"So I talked with Dr. Ginns and Barranger at NIH. I asked them what his chances would be without the transplant. What are we dealing with as far as time is concerned? What kinds of problems are we going to run into—before he dies? What can I expect? And they told me that Daniel was deteriorating very fast.

"After I got all the information that I felt I needed to help me make the decision, I looked at Daniel and I said, 'I don't know. I do not know what to do.' We were both crying." Daniel was seven years old. He asked his mother if he could die from the transplant, and if he would die without it, and after she had answered him, as she had before, he said, "I want that chance." Reba called Rappeport, and the transplant was scheduled.

Still, there were obstacles. There was yet another bleed from the esophageal varices, and another trip to Atlanta for sclerosing. And there was the information that the transplant would cost $150,000. Reba recalls Rappeport telling her, over the phone, that that was the necessary sum.

"I didn't have that kind of money," Reba says. "We didn't have any insurance. I didn't have any rich relatives.

"The community came together. They had a picture of Daniel taken and put in the paper, to explain a little about Gaucher's disease, and where everybody could see the problems. They started planning different functions. They put jars with Daniel's picture on them in different stores and restaurants and in surrounding counties—our little town couldn't have raised that much money by itself. We had car washes and cake sales, and we had auctions and donations. Then we had a Daniel Folsom Day." There was a parade and a fish fry and a softball game. "A tournament. Different teams from different counties came," paying a fee to participate. There was a trophy, which the winning team gave to Daniel, who had returned from Atlanta just in time to participate in his day, riding on the hood of the state trooper's car. "And the money was there. The hundred and fifty thousand."

Reba and Daniel flew to NIH yet again. "They did their liver function—all these tests again. And they told me that he had white spots behind his eyes. Gaucher's cells, that's all that they figured it could be, had gotten into his eyes. It hadn't affected his eyesight. Then, the fear I had was, Is he going to lose his eyesight? Is this going to cause him to go blind? And Dr. Ginns said, 'I don't know.'

"He—they—were always very honest. If they didn't know anything, they always told me, 'I don't know. All I can say is we're researching.' Dr. Ginns, he's a fantastic guy. He always had time to talk to me. He was kind of a conservative guy. And I kept picking at him, trying to get him to loosen up a little bit, because he was so straightforward. I thought then that he was starched, because that's what he reminded me of, an old starched shirt. But then he loosened up and found out that I could understand a lot of what he could tell me. And he took the time to talk to me and give me moral support. He was there to lean on. If I wanted to cry, I didn't feel embarrassed to cry in front of him. And I didn't feel that way, a lot of times, in front of the doctors."

In January, as scheduled, the Folsoms flew from the NIH to Boston, and Reba walked into Children's Hospital with a cashier's check she remembers as being for $75,000 in her hand.

"Immediately," Reba says, "everything was in order. Dr. Rappeport's whole team came in." She and Daniel arrived on a Friday, and on Saturday there were explanations of the transplantation procedure. The two Ezras, driving through a snowstorm, got there late Saturday afternoon. On Monday they went to court to get permission for young Ezra to be the donor. (Shortly after this time Massachusetts stopped requiring an actual court appearance.)

A shunt was put in Daniel's leg that day. Reba hadn't known ahead of time about the shunt, and its insertion frightened her, because "every time he was put to sleep, there was danger. They would draw blood from the artery, to measure the amount of oxygen in the blood, and his blood gases were always low. You could tell, if you watched him, how he would breathe—he also had the pressure there of the liver on his lungs and everything, too. And by this time he had Gaucher's cells in his lungs, too. So there was always that danger. Every time they'd put him to sleep, I'd have a very sick feeling myself, because I didn't know how he was going to come through it. As long as he wasn't on anesthesia very long, the danger was not so great, because he usually came right off the respirator and then straight onto oxygen. And when he came back to his room that night, he was on oxygen."

Chemotherapy started right away; there was no radiation. "It was rough, watching him go through the chemotherapy, because he was so sick at times. He had a lot of problems with retaining fluid, too. And he would go into heart failure. He'd be real swollen, and they would have to give him Lasix, the diuretic, to get rid of the fluid."

The resident, an Australian, was good with Daniel, "cutting up. And he would warn me ahead of time, like 'We're going to do this drug today or tonight' or whatever. 'And this is what's going to happen, he's going to get real sick, he could probably throw up. I want you to be prepared.'

"They would always try to give Daniel something to keep him from throwing up because of the esophageal varices, because the strain on his throat could cause them to bleed. We were always so afraid that he would bleed."

The preparatory treatment went smoothly, however. Ezra, Jr., sore but celebratory, gave his bone marrow, and Daniel "went along real good." The transplant was February 11, 1982. On March 1 Daniel passed his eighth birthday in the hospital. "He had too much fluid that day," Reba says, "and they had to give him diuretics. It was a bad birthday." Still, "Everything was going okay. He was progressing all right."

"I don't think anyone will argue," says Ginns, "that the transplant with Danny was a complete success—as far as biochemically reversing within the blood cell lines goes. We were doing experiments up in Boston in the lab there. Within thirty days after the transplant his mononuclear cells, the white cells, started coming back. We could show that his enzyme activity was completely corrected. Within thirty days."[11]

"We went ahead and transplanted him," Rappeport says, "and his counts went up, the enzyme was measured in his cells, and the iron levels were normal—supernormal, in fact—and then there was a gradual decline, over months, of the abnormal metabolic product [the stored lipid], and from that point of view things were fine. It took a number of months—seven months or more—before he really cleaned out his bone marrow. And from that scientific point of view, you showed that there could be a correction, and that these cells [lipid-laden macrophages, Gaucher's cells] stayed around for a long period of time but eventually disappeared."

Barranger says that Daniel was the first person transplanted for any lysosomal storage disease—not just for Gaucher's—and that the lessons learned from his transplant therefore apply to a whole class of diseases.[12]

Ginns says, "The life of the normal macrophage is—and of Gaucher cells should be—something like two or three months. But on repeated biopsies and aspirations, even nine months later, there were still Gaucher cells present in his marrow. Only eight to nine months later did they start really clearing out." The process may be as slow as it is because the macrophages were just not functioning anywhere near normally. There's a whole lipid burden to clean out as the new cells come in. This lipid may even be toxic, or metabolized in some way that's toxic. It's unclear."[13]

The experiment had worked. The scientific lesson of Daniel's transplant was that Gaucher's disease and other "storage diseases" were correctable and that the process, in terms of actual clinical improvement and of progress toward a cure, took longer than the positers had predicted. The resultant problem was the outcome of a paradox necessary to ethical human experimentation: Daniel had to be at death's door to justify making him the first person to undergo a potentially lethal therapy. But because he was so sick, with virtually all his organs in tenuous condition, his chances of surviving long enough to benefit from the treatment were lower than they would be for someone who needed it less. And suffering as he was from a progressive disease, the one surprise result— the slowness of returning enzyme activity—particularly worked against him.

"He was doing real well," Reba says. "He was feeling good. They had to give him red blood cells every now and then, and they still had to keep giving him the platelets."

On April 5 disaster struck. "One night," says Rappeport, referring to the night of April 4, "there was a limited number of platelets available—we had one bag, that's all there was." A hemophiliac "was eating platelets like they were going out of style.[14] It looked to me, in thinking it over, that Danny—I didn't think he was at any particular risk. At some risk, but the other child was actively bleeding." The platelets went to the child with hemophilia. "The next morning, Danny had a major bleed into his brain."

The day before, a Sunday, Reba says, "was the best day Daniel had had since he'd been in there. He was laughing with everybody. He was very outgoing with everybody. It was like, Wait a minute, something's clicked here, the kid's automatically better, he seems so different. And Dr. Rappeport came in on Sunday afternoon, because he was leaving for Israel the next morning."

Up until that day, Reba says, Daniel hadn't warmed up to Rappeport much. Rappeport had tried, she says, but Daniel hadn't responded. Rappeport "usually didn't gown up or anything, unless he had to do something to Daniel. He would just come and put his arms in through the curtain, and talk to him that way. Maybe that had something to do with it. I don't know—it was like there wasn't that one-on-one contact that much with Daniel. But anyway, he gowned up, and came in, and I said, 'Tell Dr. Rappeport the joke you just told me.' And Daniel told the joke, and just got so tickled he slapped the table, and Dr. Rappeport cracked up."

Everything, Reba thought, was fine. Young Ezra had broken his leg and, says Reba's mother, who took care of him, "He wanted to go to stay with Reba, and she had more then than she could tend to, but she took him up there."

"I said to Ezra," Reba recollects, " 'Okay, Daniel's doing so good today, you and I will go sleep at the apartment tonight.' I've never forgiven myself for that one, but then how was I to know? He had had such a good day. The nurses reassured me that if anything happened, they'd call me."

Early the next morning—about five or six, Reba says—the phone rang at the apartment, and it was the nurse who had been with Daniel all night. "Daniel has a slight nosebleed," she told Reba. "I don't think there's too much of a problem, but he's been asking for you."

Reba and young Ezra got dressed and rushed to the hospital. Daniel was sitting up, dabbing at his nose with a washcloth. "It didn't seem like a big deal, you know—the kid's nose was bleeding." But then the nurse told her that the trouble had started around four in the morning, and in the telling, Reba is angry—the nurses had promised they would call at any sign of trouble.

"And the nurse told me, after I got there, that the shunt had clotted off, and they had given him a drug to dissolve it."

Reba thinks this might have started the bleed, but Rappeport discounts this possibility, saying that the action of the anticoagulant is such that it would have left Daniel's system before the bleed started.

"I scrubbed up, naturally, and went on in with him," Reba continues, "and helped him wipe his nose when it was bleeding. They were keeping in touch with Dr. Rappeport at the time. And then the resident that was on call got there, and said he felt like he needed to pack his nose to stop the bleeding, because nothing else had helped. They'd tried to apply pressure and everything else. I guess it was about seven." Reba asked the resident why he was packing Daniel's nose. "But he was one of those kind like 'Who do you think you are? I am the doctor here, this is the patient. You're interfering.'

"Not a half hour after they packed his nose, he was out of it. He was lethargic. He didn't know anybody. He would not respond. They could tell that his pupils were dilated. And I was hysterical. Because the day before he was fine, and he had a slight nosebleed, then all of a sudden he's completely out of it.

"And that's when they called Dr. Rappeport in, and he came on in—his plane for Israel wasn't leaving till later that day. He went and checked him; he had all the reports from all the doctors. And Dr. Rappeport came out and told me, 'The neurosurgeon is coming in, and he'll be here in a few minutes.' " Reba thought that the clot that had been in Daniel's leg had moved to his brain—that is, that he had had a stroke—but Rappeport says this is not the case, that the bleed was completely separate from the clot and not, technically, a stroke. A stroke is a blockage of a blood vessel in the brain, and this was a bleeding into the tissue. The effect can be the same.

But Ginns says that the bleed could have been both a stroke and a hemorrhage, and that its occurrence could have been related directly to Gaucher's disease. "You have this problem: Is a disease you and I would also get, such as stroke or intercranial hemorrhage, due to Gaucher's disease, or is that just what is destined to happen? That's one of the questions we had with Danny: Did he have a predisposition? Did he have an aneurysm? Or was it a stroke that became hemorrhagic? Which is what I think it probably was."[15]

The neurosurgeon came out of Daniel's room and told Reba surgery was necessary to stop the bleeding. That meant keeping him under anesthesia, despite his weak lungs and heart, but there was no other choice. It also meant removing him from the laminar flow room, first for a CAT scan, which confirmed the need for the operation. Meanwhile, Rappeport left for Israel. "Brian pushed me out the door," Rappeport says.

"That hurt," Reba says. "That he left in the middle of one of the most serious situations that we had had. I had so much confidence in him. And for him to leave Daniel in that situation. I understood that the man had a personal life. But still, we needed him there. And I felt like he was betraying us by leaving. I didn't feel that we had the best anymore."

"Probably that was the hardest thing I ever saw him do," writes Ezra Folsom, Jr., of Rappeport's leaving during this crisis. "Joel was scheduled to go to Israel or somewhere in the holy land to celebrate his son's Bar mitzvah. (sp.). He didn't want to leave, but he had to. I cannot even begin to count how many times he called off and on all day from the airport and so forth. Things just didn't seem the same after all of that."

"I don't really think he wanted to go," Reba says. "He felt obligated to stay, but he had an obligation to go also, and I realize that. And now, after I've dealt with Dr. Smith and all, they were very competent. I learned that. But at that time it didn't matter to me who-all he left in charge. It just seemed like he was the only one who knew what he was doing and he's the one I wanted there.

"He could see the hurt in me, and he could see the hurt in Daniel. I could see that he was thinking, I started this, I did this to him, and now I have to walk away at a critical time. You could see the concern. I believe he had true concern there. I really do. I don't think he was ever any show, or anything. He was a gentleman."

Reba found the neurosurgeon cold, however. He would make no promises. After the operation Daniel, because of his still highly compromised immune system, was brought back to the laminar flow room rather than to an intensive care unit. His lung had collapsed, and he was intubated, attached to a respirator. His head was bandaged, his color was bad, and he was unconscious. No one knew whether he would live through the night or in what condition he might survive.

Meanwhile, Reba had contacted her family; her sister Lana Morgan and her mother, Gertie Buchanan, arrived before Ezra. "Reba," Lana says, "was beside herself." She would not let anyone touch her, shrugging off the arm her mother put around her.

Reba had also notified the NIH doctors of the bleed, "and Dr. Ginns flew up the next day to see him." "At this point," Reba says,

"I told Dr. Ginns what I thought of him, because he came in and all he really wanted was some specimens for his research. He was afraid Daniel would die before he got them. I pulled him over and told him I didn't appreciate his attitude, I didn't appreciate him coming up to get his last specimens for his research, because as far as I was concerned he didn't need those specimens. Right now all that mattered to me was for Daniel to get better. And he was like 'Wait a minute here. You know, this isn't what it's all about. I came to see about you all.' I said, 'Don't try to play up to me. It's very obvious what you want. You want your specimens. You want your stuff to do your experiments on. And see what's going on, before your patient dies.' "

Reba's reaction to Ginns was temporary—they remained friends—but her grief and fear had by now boiled into rage. "I was just mad at the world. I didn't know what was going to happen. I didn't know how I was going to deal with it if he didn't make it."

Above all, she felt her responsibility. She questioned the wisdom of having chosen the transplant, and she insisted on her right to participate in Daniel's care. She wanted him taken off morphine, so that she could assess what damage had been done. She fought with the nurses to allow her to try quieting him if he became agitated, instead of medicating him. She almost never left the hospital. Daniel's primary nurse called in her supervisor and the resident to try to calm her. Reba wasn't interested; her only concern was in trying to find and maintain life in her son.

After a few days, she got Daniel to respond: She asked him to raise a hand if he could hear her, and he did so. Once again, Reba screamed. "And everybody came running. I said to the neurosurgeon, 'I told you. I told you that he was not going to die.' So then there was hope."

But Daniel was still drugged most of the time and still intubated. When Rappeport returned from Israel (Reba remembers his absence as lasting a month; Rappeport says he was gone for two weeks), she asked if the tube couldn't be taken out. "They tried to take him off the respirator completely, but he couldn't breathe enough on his own." Rappeport said the only alternative to the respirator was a tracheotomy. "He said, 'Then we have to go through surgery again, and have to worry about the collapsed lung.' " Nevertheless, they went ahead, "and he came through it as well as could be expected, in his condition," Reba says.

Next, he hemorrhaged yet again. "One day they were trying

to put an NG [nasogastric] tube down to feed him. They needed to change it, because the tube had been in so long that it had stopped up. The nurse had tried to put it down—she didn't act too competent—and I kept warning them about the esophageal varices. I kept telling them, 'You can't keep probing down there. You're going to rupture those things.' She couldn't get the tube down—I don't know how many tubes they went through. And I kept telling them. I said, 'You're going to rupture one of those esophageal varicies.' Then they got tired of hearing that. So I stepped out of the way. But sure enough, when the resident came in, and he started poking around, and couldn't get the tube down either, he had a bleed on his hands.

"Daniel lost the full capacity of blood in his body. They were pumping in blood as fast as it was coming out. They were hand-pumping the blood into him, because it was gushing everywhere."

Rappeport rushed in; the laminar flow room was opened up. Daniel was saved once again and, a few days later, moved to a regular hospital room—with the respirator by his side. Daniel had regained speech—Reba screamed then, too—and she continued to talk to him, stimulate him, play with him. It was June. "The latter part of June. Daniel had a minor bleed after that, and in July Dr. Rappeport said it would be a good idea to go ahead and sclerose Daniel.

"Then we went into this retaining fluid again. Every time they had to up his IV, they always had to be so careful of how much fluid intake he had. Because of the heart failure he would go into.

"I kept telling them, He's retaining fluid, look how tight he's getting. They didn't seem to listen. And then he went into heart failure again. And it didn't seem that the fluid was ever going to get out of him. And during this time Dr. Rappeport came in, and I was arguing about the diuretic that he needed. And finally they did a blood test on him, and listened to his heart, found out that, yeah, he does have too much fluid. 'Get me some Lasix.'

"That's when Dr. Rappeport was standing at the foot of the bed watching him, and he looked at me and said, 'I think he's blind.'

"He said, 'Watch this,' and Dr. Rappeport would move. 'Danny, can you see me?' He'd move his head back and forth, Dr. Rappeport would, and when he'd ask him, 'Can you see me?' Daniel held his head back, looking out under the bottom part of his eyelids, really straining to see. And I think I knew that he was blind, but I didn't want to accept it. Dr. Rappeport said, 'Let me get someone up from the eye clinic to check him. I think he's blind.'

"And he was. I asked Daniel could he see me, and he said, 'No ma'am. I can't see you.' I said, 'It doesn't matter if you're blind. You can still do what you did before.' I said, 'One day your eyesight will come back.' I just encouraged him that way."

Every day, Reba worked with Daniel, helping him to write on a chalk board, assisting with physical therapy. "They never could loosen up that left side. I don't care how hard they tried, how much therapy they did, it never would loosen up. But he never lost anything but the use of his left side and his eyesight—he never lost anything mentally. He never lost that." (Daniel's blindness and paralysis were both results of his stroke, or bleed.)

Brian Smith says that once Daniel suffered the brain hemorrhage, it was clear he was doomed. "You couldn't keep him alive then. You couldn't know that right away, but you knew it a week later. The problem is that when one organ fails, and you fix that, and then another one fails, probably as a result of medication to fix the first—it's like the Dutch boy putting his finger in the dike." Smith's analogy is imprecise, but his point is clear. "There's an old intern adage that sounds cruel but is true: If you can't keep him alive when he's alive, you can't keep him alive when he's dead."

Rappeport and Ginns say the opposite. They both believe that it's possible that just as Daniel lived through catastrophe after catastrophe up to the transplant and through the events that followed, he might, with different, more consistent care than he ultimately received, have outlived his Gaucher's disease. Neither thinks the cerebral hemorrhage, or any care pertaining to it, signaled the end.

Reba says, "He was doing real well. They'd gotten him to the point where he was almost off the respirator. And then we went into the point of transferring Daniel. 'Cause here it was, August. Almost August."

Despite all the time that had passed, he still needed hospitalization, but there was no one to pay the bill.

Rappeport wanted to keep Daniel at Children's Hospital. He believes that if Daniel had remained in his care longer, he might well have averted the complication that ultimately killed him, and he might have overcome the effects of the cerebral hemorrhage. "It got better," he says. "It was getting better. Young children can get better from that kind of thing." As usual, his speech is not strongly inflected, but there is, with this sentence, a note of protestation or longing. He is sure that the transplant was effective and that in time the effects of Gaucher's disease would have been arrested and perhaps reversed. He believes that Daniel's bones would have mended and parts of his liver may have regenerated. Rappeport is also absolutely positive that he did not have the power to protect Daniel as he wished to.

Daniel had been in the hospital for seven months. "The expense," says Reba, "had gone out of—just outrageous." The cost was by now far more than the $150,000 originally estimated. "I can understand their point of view. I could understand then that this was a very big financial burden for them. But I didn't ask for that. I didn't ask for none of that to happen. Because the transplant itself would have been paid in full" had there not been the many complications, for which she was not financially prepared.

Rappeport says that one day in transplant rounds David Nathan, then head of hematology at Children's Hospital and now physician-in-chief there, announced that Daniel Folsom had to leave.

Ginns says he does not know what financial arrangements had been made.

John Barranger says that Fred Rosen, then head of the Clinical Research Center at Children's Hospital—the man with whom Barranger had first been in touch—said there was no further money available at Children's for Daniel. They were "out of support" in Boston. Barranger assumed that the Folsoms had insurance that covered their costs, until I told him otherwise, nine years later.[16]

Reba says that she gathered from Fred Rosen that the NIH had agreed to pay but had failed to live up to their promise.

John Barranger says that the NIH never would have agreed to pay for clinical care at Children's, that the only arrangement was a scientific one between himself and Rappeport.

Reba says she was "told to stay out of" the financial arrangements between the institutions, and that she did so.

David Nathan, says Rappeport, wanted to move Daniel back to Gainesville.

Lana Morgan says, "Reba found out then how little control you had over your child whenever they were in a hospital like that. I guess a hospital—Children's Hospital—I guess whenever you put your child in it, he ceases to be your child. This was the first case of Gaucher's disease that they had done a bone marrow transplant for. Maybe they wanted to keep him around for—you know, this doctor that they wanted to put to seeing after him in Gainesville had been at school with this one up at Boston." Lana does not mean Rappeport, of whom she speaks highly. Presumably she means David Nathan, since it was he who had the relationship with the Gainesville hematologist. "And I guess they thought they would get reports about everything. But it was just like Reba didn't have any say about his well-being or anything after that. I know they didn't have all the money to pay. For the hospital."

Reba says, "I could understand them. If they could get him back to Florida, Children's Medical Services would pick up the expense. But Shands had only done like one transplant and they weren't familiar with it—and I'd had bad feelings from Shands, anyway. I talked with Dr. Rappeport about it. And he was not in control of what happened—as far as moving him, or paying the bill at the hospital—but he understood where I was coming from. He realized that I wanted the best for Daniel, and he realized that possibly the best-equipped place in Florida would be Shands."

Though Reba's resentments against Shands are understandable, the staff there doesn't seem to have acted, overall, in a blameworthy manner. There were instances of tactlessness, and there may have been a lack of informativeness, but this is hard to track: doctors could not tell the Folsoms what they themselves did not know.

Rappeport says that David Nathan spoke highly of Shands to him, that Nathan said the hematologist he'd been in touch with at Shands "was wonderful" and "had agreed to oversee things, and do things in conjunction with" Children's.

Nevertheless, he says that he told David Nathan that forcing Daniel Folsom out of Children's Hospital was "not the right thing to do." He cannot remember the place or time in which he said it—he cannot recall making the statement in a formal meeting, and he does not convey that he said it with great force or insistence—but he thinks he said it twice. He says he also told Fred Rosen that he was upset about the situation with the Folsoms, and Rosen said he too was upset.

I do not have Rosen's firsthand commentary because Reba's anger at Fred Rosen's unresponsiveness to her is still so great that she refused to sign the release he required before he would talk to me about any patient. (Out of all the doctors I interviewed for this book Fred Rosen was one of only two—Peter Lariviere's ophthalmologist was the other—who required a release.)

Both Nathan and Rosen, says Rappeport, said that "the NIH had not come through as promised. The exact details of what the NIH had promised are not clear to me. Never were. But clearly I think it's fair to say that the NIH had agreed to pay in some form or other money to Children's Hospital. Whether that was going to be a supplement to the CRC [Clinical Research Center, Rosen's province] grant or it was going to be a straight cash deal, or what, I have absolutely no idea."

Again, Barranger insists an arrangement for patient care was outside the NIH's mandate, its "mission," and says, "I never tried to make such an arrangement."[17]

Nathan refused my request for an interview. Through his secretary he proposed I speak to a nurse or to the hospital's public affairs office, and stood by this suggestion although I told him—in a letter to him and orally to his secretary—that I was after an authoritative statement on a question of fiscal policy and responsibility. When I did write to a staff member of the public affairs office, asking her for Dr. Nathan's comments on who decided Daniel Folsom should be moved from Children's Hospital, I received no reply.

"It was at our expense," Reba says. "In the end, after we had gone through extended months and extended problems, we were talking about a million dollars when we left there. At that point the NIH and Children's got together and finished paying the bill," after the Folsoms left. "But no, not originally."

Apparently, there was no clearly stated and enforceable agreement worked out ahead of time about what would happen if this uninsured child, undergoing a dangerous experimental procedure—and therefore, by definition, subject to an unknown course—required medical care the cost of which exceeded the ability of his friends and family to pay.

Money was not the only issue. Reba says that at this point, after eight months at Children's, "There was too much conflict between us all. We'd been too many months of too much trouble. Everybody was on edge. I'm sure I didn't help matters any, but we couldn't get along anymore. Nobody wanted to be his nurse anymore, because he had been there so long."

(This has been a problem with other patients of Rappeport's, too. After the osteopetrotic baby had been on the bone marrow transplant unit for many months, only one nurse wanted to take care of her. The lack of improvement in the child's physical condition and the family's expression of emotional distress were strains no one else was willing to take on.)

Reba says she understood everything—she understood the expense, and she understood Daniel's bed might be needed for another patient, and she understood there were problems between her and the nurses. Also, Daniel had witnessed much of the dissension, and that was bad for him. Reba is somewhat ambivalent about whether or not she wanted to stay in Boston that August, but she says that overall, it was her first choice. "I think Dr. Rappeport—he was hearing me, he was understanding. But he couldn't do anything—his hands were tied. He wasn't in charge of everything. He was in charge of the patient, but as far as the financial part, he wasn't."

Rappeport wants doctors to be honored, and he insists that he should control his patients' treatment. And yet he did not take responsibility for as fundamental and straightforward an issue as the ability of a family to pay for the medical care he provided. Nowadays, he rails against insurance companies and hospital administrators for their say in what he's allowed to do. But in 1982, before the current era of private and public cost-limiting efforts, when financial arrangements among doctors and institutions and patients could still be made on a handshake, he was improvident and immature. He says so himself, explaining why he did not prevail in his wish to keep Daniel Folsom at Children's Hospital. "It must seem infantile," he says, describing his relationship to David Nathan, his boss. "It was part of the prolonged adolescence in which we were kept." He is referring to himself and to other doctors serving at this famous and esteemed institution. He uses the passive voice, describing the people on whose work that place's reputation rests. And he does not see, even now, how he could have acted differently. Doctors' provincialism has surfaced again: Rappeport's understanding of the balance of power is so self-referential that he cannot even imagine ways of moving outside the hierarchical status quo.

At the end of August, the Folsoms left Children's Hospital. Reba refused to take Daniel to Shands, and with the help of Barranger and Ginns arranged to have him moved instead to the hospital in Atlanta where he had been many times before for the sclerosing procedure. Rappeport did not approve of her choice. "He was very upset with me at that point," Reba says. "He felt I was making a very big mistake, which maybe I might have, I don't know, but I told him I was doing what at the time I felt was right. I said, 'I feel it's best. I do not feel comfortable taking him to Shands. I have voiced that opinion all along.' And Dr. Rappeport said, 'I think you're making a big mistake. Dr. Caplan is not a hematologist. He's not trained in bone marrow transplantation. He's a gastroenterologist.' I said, 'Yes, he is. But there's other specialists there. I'm sure he can be taken care of there.' "

The night before the move, Reba announced she was leaving and demanded copies of all Daniel's medical records. "They looked at me like I was crazy—like 'that's impossible'—but they did arrange it, and they brought it to me in boxes. A couple of boxes." Ginns and Barranger had told her she needed to bring the records with her to Atlanta.

Ginns says that Reba was calm the day they left, that she viewed the move as just one more step she had to take. He says there was no feeling of foreboding or special fear about it. But Rappeport remembers the departure as a terrible event, and in her own telling Reba was distraught. The night before leaving, she says, "I stayed up all night, afraid of what they might do as far as moving him. I don't know, I just had that fear that they might do something, and move him before the doctors from NIH could get there. By this point, there was very few talking to me. Word spread real quick that I was moving him. And everybody thought that I was acting real irresponsible. And I told them that I was doing what I felt I had to do. Dr. Barranger and Ginns got there about midnight, and they came on to the hospital and told me that they would be back at six and help make sure that we had everything ready to go. They already had all the arrangements made; all they had to do was get him out of the hospital, and we were afraid we would have to go under police escort to get him. There were a lot of ugly things being said, like, 'You don't know what you're doing. You're going to kill him.' The nurses thought I'd lost my mind."

"She wasn't always smooth," Rappeport says of Reba. "But I never found her—this isn't the right word—out of line, in any way. She had a fair amount of knowledge. She would pick up inconsistencies. And she'd find nurses that didn't know what the hell they were—well, they didn't know anything about Gaucher's disease. She did. I don't know whether that meant they were doing their job or they weren't doing their job. And certain of the nurses did have some problems because she would question us all the time. She asked a lot of hard questions. I didn't find that— I found that okay. She was fighting for her kid."

At six o'clock in the morning, Barranger and Ginns returned to the hospital. "I had him ready to go," says Reba. "We said our unfriendly farewells and we left."

One of the nurses had written a note about Reba on Daniel's chart. "They let Reba see the paper," Lana says, "that they thought she needed psychiatric help. I don't think she needed psychiatric help. She had just been through so much. All those years. It didn't affect her mind or her ability. But where it's your child and you're wanting the very best for your child and you think that somebody's trying to stand in the way of that or block it, I would be just like she was."

It is true that the strain showed in Reba: in her anger at a nurse for calling her at five instead of four for what looked like a minor symptom, for example, or in her fear that doctors opposed to her wishes might actually kidnap Daniel. The fact is, however, that she bore the unbearable for many years, and that at Children's Hospital—no matter that this was the only hope for him and a realistic one—the intensity and frequency of disasters accelerated. And in Boston, Reba was in a foreign place, among strangers. She says she found Northerners more reserved than the people she was used to. "But I always tried to respect that."

Lana sees the psychological evaluation of Reba's behavior as an insult to her sister, and Reba's conduct does seem, in the face of what she had to carry and was trying to fight off, reasonable and highly intelligible.

Daniel went to the airport in an ambulance with Ginns and a nurse. The plane was equipped as a hospital. "It was a chartered Lear jet that the NIH had arranged for us, with medical people on board, too, for everything," Reba says. "We flew for about four hours, and we got to Atlanta and they had an ambulance waiting on us to get him.

"I didn't realize until after I got him there what a big responsibility I had. Because there, I took care of him. The nurses would come in and bring his medicine; I would give it to him. They would come in and check his respirator—periodically, each shift. But as far as doing everything he needed, I was there.

"At this hospital, they had it set up where I could sleep right at the side of his bed. But he couldn't talk that loud, and if I was asleep, I couldn't hear him." Around Labor Day, her parents came to visit, and she told them that she needed a bicycle horn—"one of those little clown horns that you toot. And that way I could sleep at night, and if he needed me all he had to do is just reach out with his hand and toot his little horn.

"He was that alert. He was back to himself, he just couldn't see and he still needed the respirator now and then. They kept it right there, and kept it serviced, in case we needed to have it. We didn't have to worry to get it from intensive care. Because his lungs were messed up still, and the disease was in there, and the pressure from the liver.

"In October, Dr. Caplan said, 'Let's see if we can get him home.' And he said, 'It's time for you to start learning a little more.' And that's when the nurses started coming it, teaching me about how to regulate the IV, how to start an IV. I practiced on a nurse. They taught me how to do all these things—giving his blood. Dr. Rappeport said, Be sure the blood is irradiated. Make sure they do that to the blood before you get it. Or any of the blood products that he gets. So I made sure of that.

"We chartered us a plane and flew him home. And I was nervous as a cat. I'd been gone now almost a year, and I had the full responsibility of what happened to him on my hands." Reba knew, also, that she would have to take Daniel to Shands if there were problems. She was still unhappy about the Gainesville hospital, but right away, Daniel had to go there twice—once to be checked when he arrived home from Atlanta, and again a few days later for a transfusion. Even there, Reba inserted the IV, "because he wouldn't let the nurse. He felt more at ease if I did it. It was very hard for me to get used to doing that. But then it became like an everyday thing."

All through the fall, Reba cared for Daniel at home. "She learned to do so many of the things that the nurses are trained to do," Lana says. Daniel still had a tracheotomy tube in, to help him breathe, and a nasogastric one, through which he received most of his nourishment. Every other day, Reba drew blood, and Ezra or one of Reba's parents took it to a laboratory in Perry, the nearest large town, twenty miles away, to be checked.

And most astonishing of all, if he needed platelets or other blood products, Reba administered the transfusion. Dr. Edward

Snyder, director of Yale's blood bank, says that in his opinion, "it is imprudent at best" to transfuse blood without medical supervision and quick recourse to professional care; an adverse reaction such as shock is always possible. Though the American Association of Blood Banks publishes guidelines for the administration and supervision of blood transfusions, in many situations it is the responsibility of each dispensing institution—blood bank, clinic, or hospital—to decide how it's to be done. Snyder says the rules "should be followed at least as strictly at home as they are at the hospital," but Reba was on her own. It is another striking example, along with the one Rappeport gives of FDA requirements and the financial variability to which the Folsoms were subject, of the lack of a uniformly protective health-care policy.

Before leaving Atlanta in October, the Folsoms made an appointment to return in January. Daniel was to be sclerosed yet again, Reba says, because the Atlanta doctors said that if Daniel hemorrhaged again, "it would be a fatal bleed at that point in his life, because of all the problems that he'd had." He seemed to be in good shape at that point, though, Reba says. He'd really enjoyed Christmas, celebrated at Reba's parents. "His weight was good, his color was good," she says. But within minutes of that statement she makes another one, saying that from October on "you could see the deterioration." Nevertheless, in Atlanta doctors removed the tracheotomy tube and the NG tube. Reba does not understand why, "Because he wouldn't eat that much, because he did not have his full gag back—he could not swallow sufficiently—and lots of times he'd get strangled. At this point he's going downhill. He looks like an AIDS victim, you know, when they get in the last stages."

"Seeing someone suffer like that," Lana says, "and knowing that they will never be better, makes you a lot more able to accept their passing. Because he just withered away to nothing." His color too was terrible, yellow from liver disease, and tinged with blue from lack of oxygen.

Reba took picture after picture of Daniel. There is one of him with his brother: Daniel is leaning back, supported by pillows. His mouth is open—presumably he is trying to breathe—and as is appropriate for an eight-year-old, he is missing a couple of teeth. Veins are visible on his forehead. His eyes are directed toward the camera, but it is clear they are sightless. He is unrecognizable as the sick but still round-faced child photographed a year earlier, his brown eyes then alert, his smile slight and crooked. That boy, though, is alive in Ezra. Ezra is chubby. His cheeks are full. His mouth is firm but upturned. His hair is smoothly combed. His arm is around his dying brother, and he looks straight out from the picture, protective and knowledgeable. At the time, he was eleven.

Daniel died February 3, 1983, a little more than three weeks before his ninth birthday. One day in the last week of January, Reba says, she drew his blood. It was a Sunday morning. Ezra, Sr., took the sample to the lab, and Reba got a call. "They told me his white count was—oh, Lord—some outrageous number, it was so high. They said, 'You need to get him to the hospital, he has a terrible infection.'

"We carried him back down to Shands. And they checked it, and I thought they had everything under control. They had him on antibiotics, I thought everything was going to be okay." The next day, "He ate everything he could get his hands on, and was swallowing real well. They were going to send him home, but they were waiting for the cultures to come back on the blood they had taken the night before."

Then the doctor came in. "He said, 'He has an *E. coli* infection.' " Both Ginns and Rappeport believe the final sclerosing provoked the infection, and their paper implies it: "After several days of febrile illness following another attempt at sclerosis, he was admitted to a hospital and subsequently found to have *Escherichia coli* sepsis."[18] " 'He's not going anywhere,' " Reba quotes the doctor at Shands as saying. " 'It could be a fatal infection.' "

And yet, once again, Reba didn't really believe it. "He seemed fine on Monday." Looking back, she says, "He started dying on Tuesday. His potassium went crazy, his kidneys were not functioning right. The Lasix wouldn't even work anymore. Nothing was working. They had to give him oxygen. He started having diarrhea, and they thought he had something contagious because of the infection, so they put him in intensive care. And then the people in intensive care thought if he had something contagious, he didn't need to be in there with the rest of those very sick patients." They moved him to the seventh floor, meant for very young pediatric patients, and then they moved him to the sixth floor, where children Daniel's age were. "And he got where he wouldn't communicate. He was just out of it. It was not that they were giving him drugs. They moved him back" to intensive care.

Still, Reba did not see what was coming. "I thought we were going through some of the same things we'd always gone through, but he always pulled through. It was just like I always felt that he would always overcome it."

She kept in touch with the doctors at the NIH. Ginns was going to fly down to see if something couldn't be done. Today, he says he believes it was possible to pull Daniel through this infection, though he admits that he cannot be sure, because he wasn't there. He remembers a doctor at Shands agreeing to give Daniel respiratory and cardiac support until he could get there. He's still angry because he believes communication was poor.

Barranger agrees Daniel might have been saved, although he too says he can't be sure, because he wasn't there. And, he adds, he thinks the family did not want anything more done.

Reba called Rappeport. "I somehow felt that if I could get him back to Boston, where Dr. Rappeport was, everything was going to be okay. I had a lot of confidence in him. I really thought if I could just get him back there, that whatever was going wrong, they could fix."

Rappeport does not clearly remember the phone conversations with Reba that week, but she and Ginns say Rappeport had agreed to take Daniel back. Reba thinks perhaps Rappeport, understanding Daniel was going to die, was simply making sympathetic noises, knowing that the child could never make it to Boston, but this is inconceivable. Rappeport never lies to a patient or a patient's family about what he is able to do. In this instance, he has a vague recollection of persuading Nathan and Rosen to take Daniel back. And he, like Ginns, says he believes Daniel might have been saved. Specifically, he believes that if Daniel had remained at Children's Hospital, he might well have lived. And he reiterates his doubt about the wisdom of implementing the sclerosing procedure.

Ginns and Rappeport both talk about unsatisfactory conversations with doctors at Shands—neither of them identify, or apparently can identify, the people with whom they spoke. At almost a decade's distance, their opinion is impressionistic. Mostly, what they are expressing is frustration rather than critical analyses of their Florida colleagues. The people who had been most involved in Daniel Folsom's care did not want him to die, but they had lost control of any effort to save his life. Both Ginns and Rappeport say they would never do a transplant under these circumstances again, that one institution must be in charge throughout. And Rappeport, speaking of Shands, says, "It wasn't their mess."

Barranger says, "Would that it could have been different."

And agreeing with Ginns and Rappeport, "I think it could have been different." He believes Daniel could have survived this infection, but he gathered from the doctors at Shands—Barranger too spoke to the staff at that hospital during the final days—that in "their compassionate opinion" it was "better to let him go peacefully out. I don't agree with their decision, but I can understand their position." Doctors in Gainesville hadn't gone through "all the effort, and not just the effort, but the emotion, and the hope. They didn't have that year of real struggle to try to reverse the disease."[19]

"I didn't want to believe it was happening," Reba says of the last days. "Everybody around me knew it, but I wouldn't accept it. You could stay with him in intensive care as long as you didn't go to sleep. You had to say awake. You know, where you wouldn't be in the way." She stayed awake for two days to be with Daniel. Then he was moved yet again—first, to a regular room and finally back to intensive care. "They had him hooked up to the oxygen and to all the monitors." The family gathered. Still, Reba did not foresee the event. She sent her mother and one of her sisters to pack for her and Daniel, to go to Boston. And she herself, just for a moment, stepped out for a cup of coffee.

"And one of the doctors that had been treating Daniel stopped me, and he said, 'What would you do if Daniel died? At Shands? What would you do if we could not get him back to Boston?' " And then, Reba says, she knew. Almost simultaneously, Lana ran to her. "She says, 'You better hurry. Something's going on.' So I walked to the door," says Reba, "and I noticed there was Daniel's daddy with tears in his eyes. And it looked like it was killing him. They were trying to intubate Daniel again. And I promised Daniel, when he had gotten the tube out before, when he got the trache, that I would never let them do that to him again. Because I'd seen him suffer too long with that thing down." She sat down for a minute, and then she walked over to where the doctors and nurses were working on him. "I asked the doctor, 'What are you doing?' He said, 'Daniel stopped breathing. We're trying to put him back on the respirator.'

"I said, 'Can he breathe without it?' They said, 'No ma'am, he cannot.' 'If you put him on the machine, will he ever come off of it?' They said, 'No, he will not.' I said, 'Well, leave him alone.' I said, 'Leave him alone. He's had enough.' "

"They were so very nice to her," Lana says, "whenever they

saw that it was nearly the end. They asked her if she wanted to hold him."

"I looked at his daddy," Reba says, "and I asked him, did he want to hold him one last time? And he told me, he says, 'I wouldn't take this moment away from you for nothing in this world.' " And it is here, quoting Ezra's feeling for her, that Reba cries. In her telling of the endless ordeal that started almost as soon as Daniel was born, her feeling of isolation is ever-present. And yet when she was in Boston, she and Ezra talked on the phone every day, a fact she does not think to mention until she has finished Daniel's story. "Our phone bill was outrageous, every month," she said then. And once—during the worst crisis, when Daniel had been moved from the laminar flow room after the cerebral hemorrhage—Ezra told her he loved her. It was the only time, in all those years, he was able to say so in so many words. "Before he started to hang up that night, he says, 'I love you.' I said, 'Excuse me?' I said, 'What did you say?' He says, 'Never mind.' He said, 'You heard what I said.' "

When Daniel died, Reba says, "I think everybody on that floor could hear me. Every patient in that intensive care could. Because I was screaming at the top of my lungs. That he—had died. He died in my arms. And when he died, there was nothing left in."

Reba washed Daniel and changed his gown and left. Daniel was the first person Reba had been close to who had died. On the way home, she and Ezra talked about the funeral, "Like we wanted this one to be the pallbearer, and this song to be sung, because it was so special to him." When she got home, friends and family were there—they had come, according to local custom, to help. "But all I wanted was just to be alone. I remember going in—I didn't even take off my clothes—and laid down on top of the covers. It was cold that night, too. I just went to sleep. I didn't think I'd be able to sleep after something like that. But we were to the point where—I was—totally exhausted. All of us were. It was like every ounce of energy was gone. The fight was gone."

Ginns and Barranger came to the funeral. "They stayed and had dinner with us and everything. And then they caught a plane out that evening. That meant a lot to me. To know that they came down at their own expense and everything, and on their own time."

There was no autopsy; Reba refused both Ginns and Rappeport. They knew what he had, she said. And maybe it would be good for research—she knew it would be—but Daniel had been through enough.

Ezra Folsom and Reba are divorced now, and their farm has been sold—to relatives of Ezra's—to pay debts incurred during Daniel's illness. Both Reba and Ezra have remarried. Reba lives with Wayne Hemphill, her second husband, in a large mobile home—"a double," Reba describes it—set in a big yard. A log cabin, once Wayne's grandparents' house, sits on the same property. "Wayne offered to build me a real house, a brick house," says Reba, "but I don't need that."

Reba and Wayne are both corrections officers, each at a different state penitentiary. Reba loves her work. The facility at which she works imprisons child abusers and thieves and murderers. She likes the excitement of it, and the fact that it keeps her mind occupied. "Because if I sit idle, I think too much. I think too much about a lot of things." She is proud of the good job she does, of the physical strength she has with which to do it, and especially of her skill at counseling. "I try to show them what *good* there is out there, not just the bad." "I think I like it"—the counseling—"because I can relate to the feelings of some of these people as far as the hopelessness and the loneliness and the depression. It's like the experiences I've had."

Daniel is buried in the small cemetery in front of the church he attended. A chain link fence, erected to keep cattle out, surrounds the flat plot of land. According to the custom of the place, his picture is affixed to the gravestone. It's a painting but looks like a photograph; Reba had his school picture copied, the one from second grade. The artist rendered it almost exactly, changing only the color of the shirt he was wearing from plaid to white, and adding a tie. "An inspiration to all who knew him," the inscription on the stone reads.

Brian Smith says, "They were able to establish how fast the cells were coming in, how fast the enzyme level returned to normal, and really, the vast majority of what they were looking for. With that one patient." The experience with Daniel, he says, "has applicability to all the similar kinds of diseases and it's an example of Joel's ability to get the most out of the minimum amount of information, which is really what you have to do if you're a clinical scientist."

Rappeport talks about what has happened since Daniel died. He points to the bone marrow transplants performed on children who had storage diseases similar to Daniel's. At the end of 1990 sixteen—around the world—have been saved, at least partly as a result of knowledge gained from the treatment of Daniel Folsom.

Barranger talks about the increasing efficacy of enzyme therapy for Gaucher's disease. It does work, but it is not definitive— regular infusions are needed—and it is terribly expensive.

Ginns talks about his hopes for the research that is under way, particularly for that which will be possible if an animal model—a mouse with Gaucher's disease—can be produced.

Barranger says that because Daniel's transplant was "the first to show critical response to enzymatically competent cells from the bone marrow, it's an important thing to consider in evaluating gene therapy"; it was an early confirmation—in a human being, not a laboratory animal—that if it's possible to "get good transfer and good expression, gene therapy should be curative."[20]

"It was sad," Rappeport says, looking back, remembering the experience with Daniel, "but it was also very interesting."

It's easy to think, retrospectively, that it would have been better if Daniel had never gone through the horrors the transplant inflicted. But those horrors were not known in advance. They couldn't have been known. And so, it could not really have been otherwise. Reba had to try, for Daniel.

SEVEN

Immunity

Douglas and Barbara Schuler are like Max Perutz in that they know what they know and they know that they know it. They are assured in their expertise about deafness, the local school system, and health care. They understand a great deal about physiology, especially the immune and digestive systems, because their son Adam was born with severe combined immunodeficiency (SCID) and still has problems that are the result of this normally lethal disease and treatment for it: He is deaf as a result of an antibiotic he took before his bone marrow transplant engrafted, and he continues to have difficulty digesting food properly.

Still, Adam is normal. A bone marrow transplant saved his life, and his parents learn and teach him everything possible to maintain his health and compensate for his disabilities. I met the Schulers for the first time in New Haven, the summer Roberta was dying. They had traveled from Virginia to bring their eight-year-old son Adam to Rappeport for a checkup; I saw them in the hospital and talked to them in the playroom of the Ronald McDonald House, a beautiful, well-equipped, and well-staffed place. Barbara had recently lost a brother, and was deeply, unsentimentally understanding of what I was going through, although the purpose of my visit was to hear her family's story, with its serious difficulties. When, at Christmastime, I sent a card and told the Schulers that Roberta had died, Barbara wrote me a condolence note; we had at that time spent about three hours in each other's company.

Barbara and Doug are tall (Doug is 6'5", Barbara 5'6"), trim, even-featured, and well groomed. Adam, born July 18, 1981, is of average height. This may be because of genetic programming—Barbara thinks he will grow to be her brothers' size—but he may be shorter than would otherwise have been because of pretransplant therapy. His early years of constant illness could also play a part; children with severe combined immunodeficiency suffer from repeated, or constant, infections that are the result of having no—or virtually no—immunity and from a "failure to thrive."

Adam has his mother's blond hair, freckles, and upturned eyes. He is very active, plays soccer and baseball, and is good at them, and when my family and I visited the Schulers at home in Virginia, he was an enthusiastically demonstrative host, running through his house and across his yard in order to show my three kids around. Adam does pretty well in school, though he has trouble with math. This too may be related to the chemotherapeutic preparation for his transplant: Rappeport says one drug—methotrexate—that Adam did *not* receive, has been correlated with math deficits; it's reasonable to suppose others could have similar effects. Or it may be that his deafness makes it hard for him to learn math: "You can't learn math from a book," Barbara says. "You have to have it explained." Or perhaps it is that he just doesn't have an aptitude for the subject.

Adam is friendly and at ease with people, although during his checkup that day in New Haven, he did cry, and he sometimes removed both his hearing aids so he wouldn't have to be bothered with the conversation about him. His mother thinks he behaved as he did because the meeting with Rappeport, though it appeared relaxed, was in fact emotionally fraught. Adam had his transplant when he was a baby and cannot remember it, but his parents have conveyed to him their gratitude at the outcome.

"This is Dr. Rappeport," Barbara said to Adam, using cued speech—a combination of lip reading and hand signals based on English phonetics—to perform examining-room introductions. "He saved your life." Of course, Adam was overwhelmed. His manners are very good; he says "sir" and "ma'am" as his parents—both the children of military families—have taught him to do.

Adam does not have any brothers or sisters. Barbara and Douglas had wanted a larger family—three children, they thought—but the SCID with which Adam was born changed their plans. They were not willing to take the chance of having another baby with the same lethal disease, and although they explored adoption, and got far enough so an agency called to say a baby was available, they ultimately decided against it. Barbara went to see the little boy, and, she says, "just panicked." The Schulers had been through too much by then—seven years after Adam's birth— and had too much to cope with, to take on any more. "We didn't have another child," Barbara says, "because we needed to give all we have to this one."

She was the donor for Adam's transplant. "I wanted to do it. For one thing, Doug has this absolute fear of needles. He certainly would have done it"—"Yeah," Doug agrees, with certainty—"but hated it," Barbara says. "And in the back of my mind I felt like that if this worked, that would sort of absolve me of the sin of having been the mother—the disease, you know? I don't remember it as guilt. I remember it as feeling: If I could be the one to cure it, I sure would feel better." It did work, as T-cell-depleted haploidentical (half-matches) from parents usually do in transplants done for SCID; because the sick babies have little or no immune system (they have no T cells), the chance of failure from graft rejection is less than in other diseases. (Furthermore, when the transplant is from an HLA-identical donor, GVH is virtually unknown.)[1] Adam's hearing and digestive problems are the result of illness he suffered, and treatment he received, before the transplant gave him the T cells with which his body now fights infection.

T cells were *all* that engrafted in Adam's transplant; his body still does not produce B cells. The preparation for his transplant did not include an agent—irradiation or drugs—to destroy the pluripotent stem cell, because it wasn't necessary to do so. In SCID, there is no malignancy to treat, nor is there a malfunctioning of a blood component, as is true, for example, in children suffering from Wiskott-Aldrich syndrome, who, in addition to lacking fully functional T cells, have incompetent platelets. Adam had a functioning hematopoietic system; his red cells and platelets were fine—he wasn't anemic, nor was he bleeding—and he had granulocytes, too, enabling him to fight some kinds of infections.

"But granulocytes can't do everything," Brian Smith says. Without them, "You don't do well with viruses at all. So you get cytomegalovirus, and you die, and that kind of thing. You also, to make the granulocytes work well against everything, need antibody around. Which is made by the B cells. So probably if you were a sponge—if you had a more primitive, from an evolutionary point of view, defense system—you could get away with just granulocytes." In a sense, Smith says, "aplastic anemia is the reverse of SCID. Because patients with aplastic anemia are missing the hematopoietic arm of the system—red cells, granulocytes, monocytes, platelets." But they have the whole lymphoid system, "the exquisitely specific, wonderful, detailed immune system that we all know and love." He is, as usual, cheerfully sardonic. The unknowns and surprises of the immune system are, as they have been for years, the day-in, day-out challenges, headaches, and fears of his intellectual and work life.

Barbara was nineteen and Doug twenty-three when they were married, and Adam was born six years later. "In hindsight," Barbara says, and Doug agrees, "I'm awfully glad we waited to have a baby. I don't know if a young marriage would have lasted. Because the next couple of years," following Adam's birth, "were just pure hell."

When he was born, he seemed completely normal. Perfect. "When he was about four months of age," Barbara says, "he got what they call a perineal abscess—just a little infection, around his bottom. It was no big deal: They told us over the phone what to buy and do for it. And we did that, and nothing happened, and nothing happened, and it would not go away. It got to the point they had to do some minor surgery on it. And after that it just got massively infected and—the only way I could describe it, is it looked like they had split a shrimp down the back—and you know how it puffs out? That's what his rear end did."

It went from bad to worse, Barbara says, and soon—when Adam was about six months old—their pediatrician said, "It's time we started looking." The doctor had a reason for worrying, aside from Adam's symptoms. Ten years earlier, Barbara's infant nephew had died one day after having been diagnosed with SCID.

"Adam looked fine at this point. In fact, my sister kept saying, 'He doesn't have it,' because her son had looked so ill." But tests at the local hospital showed something was wrong, and the Schulers' pediatrician referred them to an immunologist in Washington. He made the definitive diagnosis, and suggested doing a thymus implant. It took three months for the necessary fetal tissue to become available, however, because the Catholic hospital with which the immunologist was affiliated would allow him to use only spontaneously aborted fetuses.

"During that time," Barbara says, "Adam almost died. He developed thrush so bad that it was in his mouth, his whole esophagus." Thrush is a fungal infection that causes pain and swelling. "He could hardly swallow. The only thing that was keeping him alive at that time was the fact that he was being breast-fed." He was able to nurse, and he received some immunity from his mother. Nevertheless, he was down from 19 pounds to 11. Barbara's sister, experienced with doctors, told her that Adam was dying, that things were taking too long, that she had to push the doctors. "She said, 'You have got to scream and rave.' I had not been burned at that time yet by a doctor. She'd been burned a couple times."

Barbara wrote a letter to the Washington immunologist, pressing him to act, but a thymus became available before he received the letter, and the implant was done. "They were trying it," Barbara says, "because it was a very benign procedure. They take a thymus and they literally chop it up and encase it in a little capsule and they stick it in your abdomen, hoping that—"

"It would trigger things," Doug says, "as far as the immune system going into action—the thymus putting out the right hormone or whatever to activate the cells."

"To grow T cells," Brian Smith explains, "and make them smart—to educate them—they need to come out of the bone marrow, and go into the thymus, that thing sitting in your neck, and then wander on. And that's when they get educated. Now, you and I don't have much of a thymus left. In fact, by the time we're about thirteen, fourteen, fifteen there isn't much of a thymus left. But you don't need it—probably, most of the time—after you're that age." By then, "You've already educated most of your cells to all of those horrible things that all your friends gave you when you were a kid."

It isn't all that simple, he goes on to say, because after a bone marrow transplant, even in an adult, even if the marrow was T-cell-depleted, "you do redevelop T-cell function afterward. It could be that the reason for this is that the person you get the bone marrow from had all these T cells that were already educated," even the immature ones that would remain after T-cell depletion, "and so you weren't really redeveloping it from scratch." On the other hand, "Some theories of graft-versus-host disease—particularly chronic graft-versus-host disease," the type Peter Lariviere suffered from for so long, "say that the problem is you can't educate your T cells. They remain stupid, they never become tolerant of you. And so they sit there both being ineffective and attacking you."

In any case, the thymus implant "had no effect," Barbara says. The next step was a bone marrow transplant, about which the Schulers, despite Barbara's sister's experience, knew nothing. At that time, because the baby died so quickly, the family hadn't had a chance to investigate bone marrow transplantation. And of course the procedure was much newer and riskier in the early 1970s than it was ten years later, although the first successful bone marrow transplant—on a boy from Connecticut, transplanted in Minnesota—was done in 1968.[2]

When Matthew died in 1972, his doctors said the experience was a fluke—that Barbara's sister and brother-in-law both had a recessive gene, resulting in Matthew's having an autosomal disease, and that SCID shouldn't repeat itself. If their remarks seem uninformed as well as uninformative today, it's not only because doctors now speak with greater care, presumably largely in response to malpractice suits, but also—and this is more important—because the continuing explosion of knowledge in molecular biology and genetics had barely begun two decades ago. Even doctors alert enough to diagnose SCID and suggest a bone marrow transplant may not have known either the likelihood of its happening again in the same family or the probability of its having occurred in the past.

"If you knew everything," says the immunologist Fred Rosen, "you could predict everything . . . and presumably prevent everything. But we don't know that much. We're living through a remarkable two decades, where the explosion of knowledge has just become fabulous. And you realize you've just scratched the surface. There's so much more to know."

"The characteristics of severe combined immunodeficiency," Rappeport says, "have been expanded and expanded and expanded. So that some of the children have no lymphocytes. Some of them have lymphocytes that don't work. Some of them have lymphocytes that have abnormal molecules or absences of molecules." So

that once again, like leukemia and myelodysplasia and aplastic anemia, SCID is "a very heterogeneous group of diseases."

After it became apparent Adam was sick, another family memory, not seen as significant until then, added to the precision of the
diagnosis: a great-aunt of Barbara's on her mother's side had had
two children, both boys, who died in infancy of pneumonia. Retrospectively it seemed clear that they too had had SCID. Of the
many forms of the disease—Rappeport says there are about fifteen
genetic variations—one is X-linked, and this is apparently the type
Adam had. Fred Rosen says he can't be sure, but thinks so. "There's
no way to know. We don't know what the defect is in X-linked.
The gene has been mapped, approximately. But we're not certain
of what the gene defect is."

"I had three healthy brothers," Barbara says. "And my mom
had two brothers. I remember my mom had guilt that it had hit her
daughters." This is an additional irrational curse of genetic disease,
especially that which is carried from mother to son. Although Barbara's mother was obviously not in any way at fault for what happened to her grandsons, she bore the entirely unjust burden of
feeling that she was to blame.

And at this time—1991—there is no way for a family to avert
X-linked SCID. (Rappeport says a prenatal test for another form—
ADA deficiency—is available.) Fred Rosen says there isn't yet a
reliable test for carriers.[3] Even if there were, the rarity of the
disease makes it unlikely that there would be widespread screening.
A family's first indication is a child actually born with the disease,
and today the only way to be sure a second won't follow is to avoid
conception.

In this way SCID is—currently—even more of a familial affliction than Wiskott-Aldrich syndrome, where testing of both carriers and fetuses is available. If Adam did have a sister, she would
not be able to achieve the relative peace of mind available to Beverly
Hough. "I often think I would like a little girl," Barbara Schuler
says. "In *addition* to Adam." But she is firm that this is not to be.

Despite Barbara's healthy brothers and uncles, the Schulers'
decision to limit their family is, with the state of today's knowledge,
both responsible and intelligible.

The immunologist in Washington told the Schulers that a
bone marrow transplant was the last resort, that it was very difficult, and that the prognosis was not good "with a bone marrow

transplant, at that time," Douglas says. Less than ten years after Adam's experience, bone marrow transplants are successful standard treatment for SCID, with long-term survival estimated at 60 to 70 percent, even if the donor and recipient are only an HLA half-match.[4]

"I remember being very afraid of it," Barbara says. "And yet I remember thinking in my heart that it was the only thing. We saw him dying before our eyes. And having had my nephew die, I *knew* that that happened if you did nothing, if you were not able to do anything."

"I remember questioning it a little bit," says Doug. "I went to get a book on it. And of course once we got up there [to Boston] and started talking to people, it was quite obvious that there was no other choice. Plus, we knew—I guess from David, the boy in the bubble—and again, it's common sense—if your body cannot fight infections and you already have all these infections, you're doomed. You can't put him in the bubble then, it's too late, because he's already exposed. So the only choice at that point was to give him an immune system, and the only way you can give him an immune system is with the transplant. So logically, this was our only choice."

"We also had our pediatrician at home," Barbara says, "who is second in our hearts only to Joel. Dr. Popish was saying the same thing, that this is what you have to do. So I remember questioning, having fears at this point as far as having to do it, but I remember feeling it had to be done. And the perineal abscess was still flaring up. That was a constant visual reminder. He had to take sitz baths twenty minutes long every two hours, and by the time you sat there for half an hour, and got him out and dried him off, it was time to get back in there. That was just a constant thing."

"Plus which," says Doug, "he continues to eat, and he continues to lose weight. What do you do? He's just wasting away in front of your eyes."

The Schulers, like other loving parents, have thick albums full of snapshots. Theirs show just what they've described: at first, a healthy baby, next to a big plastic apple. Then a wan, thinner Adam; Barbara says they lied about his age then, so as not to have to explain to strangers. There's a picture of Adam having a sitz bath in the kitchen sink; here, his ribs show. And there's another where his skin is visibly wrinkled, a result of the weight he's lost. He looks like a victim of that other, similar disease, then basically unheard of, now much better known than his affliction, and far, far more widespread: AIDS. The acronyms are similar for good reason. In fact, Fred Rosen says, "without defining SCIDS, AIDS never would have been known."

Right before the Schulers went to Boston for the transplant, they decided to have Adam baptized. Barbara, though she had not recently practiced her religion, had been raised a Catholic, and particularly wanted the baptism. The priest she called, however, refused her. She was not a member of his congregation, he told her, and he would not do it. It was the end of Barbara's affiliation with Catholicism. The Schulers then called a Presbyterian minister they knew slightly, and he offered to come over immediately and baptize the baby. Barbara and Doug assured him the next day would do, and Adam was baptized then. Of course, this story isn't a condemnation of Catholicism or an endorsement of Presbyterianism; it's an example of the variability of people's characters in any profession. The Schulers dealt also with their share of both the good and bad among doctors and nurses during Adam's transplant.

"We had one resident who was a bozo," Doug says. "I won't mention his name. As a matter of fact, I don't remember his name." It's sort of the tomb of the unknown soldier: This person, or one just like him, could have served a rotation during anybody's long hospitalization. "He came in one day, and he was being his little egotistical self," Doug says. "He was treating me like dirt, he was treating Adam like dirt, and I grabbed him, and I said, 'You're going to do it the way I want it done, or I'm going to throw you out this window right here.' " Quoting himself, Douglas employs his usual calm, uninflected tone. He is a policeman—at the time of Adam's transplant, he was a supervisor on the evening shift, and he's now a crime prevention officer—and he has a measured, just way of speaking and a manner that, combined with his size, convinces the listener both that he is right and that he will prevail.

"He left," Doug says of the offending doctor, "and they sent somebody else in. And then—oh, boy—they placated the hell out of me. And I said, 'I don't care. This guy came in here like he was God, and acted like I didn't know what I was talking about.' I grabbed him and threatened to throw him out the window. And I would've, too. I don't know if I would've or not. But damn, I was mad."

This incident took place almost at the end of Adam's very long hospitalization. "After eight months of this," Barbara says, "you learn a little bit about it. Plus, you're a parent, you're with this kid all the time, and you get a feel. . . ." Barbara's words contain an echo of Rappeport on the subject of Reba Folsom: her problems with nurses stemmed from her vigilance and her expertise.

There was one nurse, for instance, says Barbara, who "hooked up a whole IV line full of air and started it, before we said, 'You—have—not—primed—the—line.'" And another, "a new little nurse—we frightened her, and yet, you know, your kid is the primary thing. She was brand new, they were just training her, and she kept leaving needles on the bed, and with a two-year-old child here, you cannot do that. She was nervous and new, and she kept making dangerous mistakes. We went to our head nurse and said, 'We're sorry, we cannot have that young girl. Let her learn on somebody else.' And they said fine, and they did."

The Schulers say they encountered more ignorance and ineptitude on the part of the nurses than they did with the doctors, but they agree that most of the nurses were excellent. The Schulers became friends with some of them. They were happy with nearly all the doctors, too. They remember one man, himself the father of a young child, who used to sit with Adam in the evenings, just to be with him and offer his company.

On the other hand, there was a surgeon who, when telling them Adam would need a colostomy, neglected to mention that it was temporary. "And I thought," Barbara says, "Gee. He's going to be deaf, he's going to have a bag—what kind of a life, what kind of an adolescent is he going to be? It wasn't until a week later that he said, 'You realize I'm talking for six months.' And I could have slugged him. I realize it wasn't his fault. But it would have made a big difference to me if he'd said that in the first place."

At this point the Schulers were staying in an apartment near the hospital. They had originally planned for Barbara to stay in Boston with Adam and for Douglas to return home to his job. But a young doctor, right off, said, "This takes two. If you can possibly manage it, this takes two." And Barbara and Doug agree, it did. "Doug was able to get a leave of absence from work," Barbara says, "and stayed the whole time. Initially our plan had been to go up, and Doug would stay two weeks, right over the transplant, and then leave. We got up there, and they didn't do the transplant for about two months because of all the infections, and I could not have handled it by myself. The stress was such that I would—we took turns sleeping late. And if I slept late, Doug would go over in the morning and handle Adam, and then I'd get up at noon, and Doug would come home and go back to bed. That was the only—you could escape it when you were asleep. We ate a lot. And when we went out to eat we drank too much." Doug disputes the latter.

The apartment was terrible, Doug says. "No furniture. There were a couple of chairs, a couple of beds. There was a TV set with coat hangers as an antenna."

"We had to put the bed—a metal-frame bed—in little buckets, little bowls of water, to keep the roaches off," Barbara says. "And then they dropped off the ceiling. I mean, it was bad."

The transplant was on October 30, 1982, when Adam was fifteen and a half months old. Up until then, Barbara says, "there was a lot of waiting, and a lot of watching him get, you know—smaller. We kept him away from people. At this point we knew that he was ill, and he certainly wasn't allowed around children. We went to families" when visiting in Virginia, before going to Boston for the transplant. "If the adults weren't sick, we would visit with families."

"We didn't even do that too much," Doug says.

"It was just a lot of waiting," says Barbara.

Waiting, they say, was all along, through everything, the hardest part.

After the decision to try for a bone marrow transplant was made, they flew to Boston and spent two weeks there for tests and evaluation. "They did a lot of blood work," Doug says. "He was so small and so malnourished and everything that every time he got blood taken, nobody could get a vein. You couldn't just take it out of his arms. They had to stick him in the jugular vein, in the neck. And that was very traumatic. But it got to the point where it was fairly routine, to do jugular sticks on him."

Barbara says Adam "didn't have a lot of energy," but wasn't actually listless. He developed normally and could walk at fourteen months. "I vividly remember him walking down on Division 20 [the Children's Hospital floor on which the evaluation was being done] when he was fourteen months. He weighed 11 pounds, and he's walking down the floor and his diaper dropped off, and I just sat there and cried. He was this little, tiny, emaciated guy."

"He was weak," Doug says. "I remember one of the doctors dictating to his machine, and saying he was in stage 3 of malnutrition. It's something to do with the disease. For some reason, the body evidently doesn't absorb things like it should. But I remember Barbara blaming herself for it then."

"I nursed him until the day they put him in the sterile room. Then I stopped," Barbara says. "And that was traumatic for me. Because all along I felt at least he was getting some immunities. You know, that was sort of my security blanket. I felt like, shoot, we're taking away the one thing that he has that everybody has said has maybe helped him. But it wasn't sterile, so they had to stop that."

After the initial evaluation in Boston, the Schulers had flown home to wait until a bed became available. That happened sooner than they'd thought it would, because, says Doug, another bone marrow transplant patient died. The Schulers flew back again two weeks later, and the grueling process began. Not only was it weeks before Adam's infections cleared enough for the transplant to be possible, but there wasn't a take—an engraftment—until nearly two months after Barbara's marrow was infused.

"He didn't engraft," Barbara says. "We got the first news, as far as engraftment, on December 23." The probable reason for the delayed engraftment was that Barbara's marrow was T-cell-depleted before it was administered to Adam. Though the baby needed T cells, he would have to rely on those that would develop from precursors. Barbara's *mature* T cells could have caused lethal GVH, because she and her son were genetically only a half-match, as is usual between parent and child.

In March 1983 Adam was discharged from the hospital. The Schulers had made a lot of friends, and been friends to other people. They never felt the need of a formal support group and had trouble recalling the psychologist who was in charge of one, because they formed their own ties with other parents caring for their children in adjoining and nearby rooms. When they arrived, parents of a child being transplanted for osteopetrosis "helped us out a little bit," Doug says. "They said you gotta do this, you gotta do that, you can't have that put through the autoclave [the sterilizer] and that helped. Having someone show you the ropes a little bit. And once you're there awhile, you learn the ropes, and I think we were helpful for other people."

The Schulers are still close to the family of the child who had osteopetrosis. This child, a boy, has survived. His aunt was the donor. Several years after the experience they shared, the Schulers visited the other family. The little boy "had three bone marrow transplants before it took. He's a year younger than Adam and is about twenty-four inches tall." Unlike Adam, he was irradiated. "The radiation and what have you, they feel, has obviously done something to his growth. And caused cancer in him also." He has been treated for lymphoma. "And he is blind." Osteopetrosis itself did that; with this boy, the disease had progressed far enough to destroy his eyesight before the transplant could halt it.

It was easier for the Schulers to talk with people going through the same thing, hour by hour and day by day, than it was to explain things to even the most loving family, hundreds of miles away. The parents of other children receiving bone marrow transplants knew what the counts meant, knew how Hickman lines worked, understood the "roller-coaster"—a universally employed metaphor—nature of the process. Allusions were quickly picked up; empathy was the order of the day.

Getting out of the hospital was a euphoric experience for the Schulers. "That was just the best day of our lives, of course," Barbara says.

"I mean we were in that damn hospital forever," Doug adds.

Instead of returning immediately to Virginia, they took Adam to a different, only slightly better apartment than the roach-infested place in which they'd stayed at first. Rappeport wanted to keep an eye on him for a while.

"And before we left, Joel said, 'You know, we really need to go have his hearing checked.' We had no inkling at all there was a problem—but since he'd been on the amikacin" there was reason for concern, but "after all this time Doug and I said, 'No, this is enough, his hearing's fine, we're going home.' And Joel said, 'Hmm, just let's—you know . . .' " This is the way Rappeport often talks, accompanying his few words with shrugs and grimaces. "Well," Barbara goes on, "we had it checked, and Adam didn't respond to a thing. But he was just so crazy for being out of this room for the first time in so long, he was just a wild little baby, and the woman came out and said, 'Your son has a profound hearing loss.' And we said, 'No, he doesn't. He's been in a bubble for so long, and he hasn't seen people's mouths.' And you could see the look in this woman's eyes: 'I've got these crazy parents.' "

It was not irrational for Barbara to draw this incorrect conclusion. In the hospital, Adam had lost at least one other attribute of normalcy. "They had to have a behavioral psychologist reteach Adam to eat. It had been so long since he had eaten anything orally;

everything had been done by IV. We'd put food in front of him, and he would play with it. He had absolutely no remembrance or connection or whatever." The nurses pulled down the shades, turned off the TV, and applauded every time Adam put food in his mouth, until he had the habit back again. No wonder Barbara thought he might not act like a hearing person and yet still be one.

"We went back and told Joel that they say he's deaf, but he's fine. And we left the hospital, and we got back to our apartment, and we'd gotten him a little toy that you wind up, and it ran across the linoleum floor making noise."

"It was a train," Doug says. "A little locomotive."

"It made this loud, loud noise," Barbara says. "And Adam was sitting on the floor with his back to us, and we wound that up and put it down, and he didn't look up until it passed him, and Doug and I said, 'This child is deaf.' And so the best day of our lives turned into—I felt like somebody was upstairs with a big two-by-four, just batting, you know." Because of the hearing loss, "they stopped the amikacin, and two days after that his bottom just went crazy, because of the infection." It was then that surgeons performed the colostomy.

"We found out Adam was deaf, and then two days later this doctor was talking, talking, talking, and 'By the way, you know he has to have a colostomy.' Well, I just . . ."

"Lost it?" says Doug.

"It was true. I just thought, you've got to be kidding." To have come so far, Barbara says, to have reached a point where it looked as if everything would be all right, and then to learn of the handicaps they, with Adam, must face . . .

Adam's deafness is the result of the antibiotic he took for his persistent rectal infection. "We were still battling this perineal abscess," Barbara goes on. "Even though he was engrafting, the infection was still flaring up and down, and they were sending cultures here and there trying to determine what it was. They found out it was an atypical mycobacteria, and started treating it with amikacin. And other things. But I remember the amikacin."

Because it was the culprit in Adam's hearing loss.

"They had told us," Barbara says, "that it could affect his hearing or his kidneys. And they checked—daily—these kidney levels. And it never affected his kidneys. It was extremely unusual that it affected his hearing without affecting his kidneys. It was just one of those fluky things. But that infection was such a problem—

we'd battled it for almost two years, and it was still going strong. And so something had to be done about it."

As it turned out, Barbara said, the colostomy was not traumatic after all. Dealing with a colostomy bag was easier than dealing with diarrhea, and in six months, with the infection finally cleared, that particular part of the ordeal was over. The Schulers by then were home—they'd left for Virginia the end of April—though for several months Barbara and Adam flew to Boston often so he could be checked.

"It was frustrating when we got home," Douglas says, "because it was almost two years before he could have contact with other kids."

"I remember giving him a bath," Barbara says, "and crying and crying, calling my mother because I was so housebound." Her mother, who then ran cosmetics stores, gave Barbara a job, working from ten to three and Saturdays. "I was underworked and overpaid," Barbara said of her outside employment. "My mother would disagree, but I think she lost money on the deal." Doug worked nights, so that a parent could always be with Adam. "We didn't want to hire someone," Barbara says. "He had a colostomy, and a hearing problem." Adam's parents entertained him, but they worried about "whether he would trust people, whether he would just turn out a strange little person—he went through a lot of bizarre stuff," Barbara says.

She thinks now Adam is emotionally normal—sensitive, but then so is she—"except for in some social skills, he's about three years behind. During those crucial years when we all develop so much, Adam was on the other side of the chain link fence from everybody else." This isn't a metaphorical statement; Barbara is referring to the years that Adam, because of the risk of infection, couldn't be allowed to play with other children, and to his longing to do so. "There were kids next door. And Adam would go out and cling to the chain link fence. And just watch these children. It was like—little knives. In your back. In your heart. It was real hard."

Doug is astonished that Barbara doesn't mention Adam's deafness as a factor in his social development. She immediately agrees it's an important element, and quotes Helen Keller: "Blindness cuts you off from things, deafness from people." It's a vivid explanation of the feelings of the osteopetrotic baby's parents, who said they were willing to accept blindness in their child, but not so sure of their capacity to handle one who was also deaf. Barbara says Adam has trouble in groups, where he has to "work much harder to fit in, to understand. That has to have affected him, he has to have learned from it, but he couldn't tell you what."

Adam has not yet learned to restrict his diet, the cause of his second major set of physical problems. Adam cannot digest sugars; he is intolerant of lactose, sucrose, dextrose, and fructose. He is not supposed to have milk or milk products, candies or cookies or cakes, any processed food that contains sugar—fish sticks, for example, are off-limits, and nearly all breads—and the vast majority of fruits and vegetables. String beans and carrots, for example, disagree with him. He can have red meat, chicken and fish, lettuce, Brussels sprouts, pita bread, and potatoes. He would like to have corn on the cob, candy, and ice cream, and sometimes he does eat these foods. He's not at risk of going into shock, or having some other dangerous reaction, but his body neither retains nor absorbs the proscribed foods normally. Instead, if he eats something he shouldn't, he has gas and diarrhea for a day or two afterward. The way in which the problem is a major nuisance and embarrassment is also a result of Adam's repeated, massive, persistent rectal infections. Though they are now a thing of the past, they damaged his sphincter muscle so that he can't control the diarrhea; he has frequent accidents in school and in public.

No one can say for sure that the transplant caused this food intolerance or that it derives from SCID, but, says Barbara, "When I ask, the answer I get is 'That's a good question.' I just can't believe the human body can go through so much and not have something go wrong." In any case, there's apparently nothing to be done about it except hope it will go away. That's a possibility, but one in which Barbara places no stock. If it's an allergy, Doug says, Adam may outgrow it. But Barbara thinks it's an enzyme deficiency, and that therefore the problem is here to stay. "You can see who's the optimist," she says. "But it was supposed to be okay when he was six. Now, out of self-preservation, I've decided this is how it's going to be. The gastroenterologist in New Haven said even if they find out what's wrong, they can't fix it."

Barbara doesn't have the heart to deny Adam everything he likes to eat. He's a growing boy. It's hard to fill him up with only the things he should have, and when she lets him have dessert, he hugs her and thanks her. Eating what he shouldn't doesn't make him feel sick or uncomfortable, so in the summer, when cleaning up after him is her burden and not the school's, and when she is home rather than at her ten-month-a-year school-system job, she gives him leeway. Still, she hopes that soon he'll take positive control of his own eating habits. "What's acceptable at three isn't acceptable at nine. I keep thinking when he gets older, kids will get to him, and it will right itself. Maybe it will take the cute little girl sitting next to him or the bully. It sounds cruel but I don't mean it that way. But he knows Mom and Dad will love him anyway."

The Schulers moved after the transplant. Barbara says she knows a lot of people who did this, and lists them by name, all families whose children were stricken, often with rare diseases, and always with ones that, without a transplant, would surely have killed them. In every instance she mentions, I can remember terrible trauma additional to that of the primary blow. There's the child who had osteopetrosis and now, at eight, is blind and only two feet tall. There's the boy whose severe GVH has cost him his teeth and the ability to move his body properly; he's in a wheelchair. There's the teenage girl who's had GVH but, aside from some special eye care, is fine. When she was sick, though, one of her brothers, of elementary school age, used to say that he hoped he'd get hit by a car, because if his sister died, he wanted to, too. And another brother, her donor, had a breakdown that required repeated hospitalizations.

Barbara says she's convinced that people move after a transplant to reestablish control over their lives. "For so long, doctors told us when he could eat. People told us when to change his diapers. I remember feeling at the time almost in people's way, of them taking care of my child. Although they certainly wanted us there. But people literally told you when to eat, and when to brush his teeth."

As Adam gets older and the world beyond his family gets more important to him, the Schulers' concerns grow. Some children go out of their way to be kind to Adam and help him, but others are cruel. Some teachers are sarcastic and negative. One teacher laughed at Adam for making mistakes. "He didn't notice, but other kids did." It is difficult to get the help to which Barbara and Douglas know Adam is entitled, and the materials that he needs. His teacher speaks into an audio trainer—a microphone beamed to Adam's hearing aids—but it took years for the school system to install in his classroom a carpet to reduce reverberations from linoleum floors and cinderblock walls—thus maximizing Adam's chances of using whatever hearing he has—though they'd agreed to it and the Schulers offered to pay for it and move it, if necessary.

Barbara and Doug have had to fight to have the degree of Adam's handicap acknowledged and dealt with as they wish. They appear to know *everything* about hearing loss and methods of communication for and with the deaf. "Unaided," Barbara says, "he can hear 70 decibels." Normal speech, Barbara explains, is about 30 to 35 decibels. By contrast, "ninety is like a jet. If you put your mouth up to Adam's ear and yell, he can hear it. With his hearing aids, it's 40 decibels. He can hear speech, but he can't understand it, because of nerve damage. Life is much easier when he can wear his aids." But he still has frequent ear infections—"back to back for a year and a half, then he seems to get over them, then he gets another"—and fluid in his ears. (Brian Smith says some of this may be because the transplant was partial; Adam's lack of B cells means his T cells don't work optimally against infection.) These complications prevent him from wearing his hearing aids and decrease his ability to hear under any circumstances. "Right now," Barbara says, speaking at the end of the summer before Adam is to start fourth grade, "he can hear 120 decibels, and even aided it can't be under 40, so he can't hear." If he understands speech, it's because he's lip-reading. The school system can't understand that." It's easy to see why. Adam's speech is close to normal, and his sociability and energy and sense of humor and general air of happy adjustment make it easy to think, as both goodwill and laziness could incline an administrator to do, that everything is fine.

"He's bright," Barbara says. "Not gifted. But bright." Nevertheless, his grades slipped the previous year, as academic work became the dominant part of the curriculum. The average deaf person, Douglas says, reads at the fourth-grade level. He says deaf children dependent on sign language usually cannot communicate well with their fathers, who are not with them enough to learn fluently what is essentially a foreign language. The Schulers do not want Adam in special education classes. They are intent on keeping him in the hearing world—their world. Some hearing families with a deaf child depend on lip reading alone, but the Schulers think that would be too limiting for Adam. That is why they use cued speech, which, though it has hand signals, is not sign language. Because cued speech is based on phonetics, it is closer to spoken language than is conventional sign language. In sign language, for example,

says Barbara, you cannot rhyme. And the sign for temple, syna-
gogue, and church is the same—that is, in sign language they are
the same word. When she introduced my husband and children to
Adam, Barbara points out, she could cue the syllables of their
difficult last name, and he could immediately say it aloud. Sign
language, the Schulers say, takes years to learn. They were able to
start using cued speech right away.

The Schulers insist the school provide speech therapy, and a
"hearing itinerant teacher"—a specialist who comes into the classroom. They worried all summer about whether they'd persuade the
school to provide the additional help Adam needs, but in October,
Barbara writes to tell me that the special education board has agreed
to provide an interpreter, trained in cued speech, to tell Adam what
the regular classroom teacher, and the other children, are saying.
The board agreed, she says, because Adam's chronic ear infections
so often prevent him from wearing his hearing aids:

> Right now we are fighting a fungal infection in the rt. ear, and a
> middle-ear infection in the left. The frustrating part is that the
> antibiotic needed for the m.e. infec. causes the fungal infec. Sounds
> familiar, doesn't it?
>   "Great News!" [Doug, who's been going to college in addition
> to his job, has finished school.] As of Tues. he is a free man (if you
> don't count his wife, son, house, bills, etc. . . .)

"There was a time," Barbara said to me when we first met,
telling me the beginning of Adam's story, "when I just thought,
'Oh, God, let him live. I'll never say a foul word. I'll never get
angry again.' There are days, now, when I'd sell him for a dime.
And I'm glad it's gotten to the point where you can worry about the
car breaking down, and the refrigerator breaking down, although
we can usually put it in perspective: Okay, you're mad, but just
remember, for this we can whip out the Mastercard. And we remember when Adam was sick, you just think if it was something
where you could give your house or your arm or anything. And
now most of our problems are things you can solve. Adam's come
through an awful lot. Yes, he's a nice little boy.

"It's because we've worked so hard, not because it doesn't take
any work."

In August 1990 the troop buildup that precedes what is to be
the Gulf War has just begun. The Virginia town in which the

Schulers live is a suburb of Norfolk, and jet noise is almost constant. It does not usually trouble Barbara and Doug. Because of their fathers' occupations they have always lived on or near military installations. Barbara says she's accustomed to thinking of the noise of the planes as "the sound of peace." But at this time Barbara and Doug are worried, because many of their relatives and friends are being sent to the Middle East, or expect to be soon. The concern shows on Barbara's sensitive face.

The Schulers' house, in a neighborhood of quiet streets, is orderly and peaceful. They've installed a small decorative pond in the backyard, and Barbara and Douglas and I sit by it, glasses of iced tea in our hands, talking about Adam and all the hard and measured decisions they've made for and because of him.

Barbara does most of the talking, and Doug says this is because they decided ahead of time that it would be easier if one of them is the spokesperson. But I think perhaps he wants her to tell the story because he so admires her part in it. It is Barbara, Douglas says, who did most of the research on ways to help the hearing-impaired. It is Barbara who vacuumed the house constantly, and scrubbed it, after the transplant. "And I'm not that kind of a house-keeper," Barbara says.

Doug did his share, and it's clear he still does. The most striking thing about the Schulers, however, is that although nearly all we talk about is Adam, they do not seem preoccupied with him or overly absorbed in him. I know they feel, as does everyone in similar circumstances, that fate's been unintelligibly cruel. But their composure and openness is constant. They never act injured. The difficulties that exist must be dealt with, that's all.

EIGHT

≈≈≈≈

New
Prospects

When Patrick Thompson and Jane Morse became Rappeport's patients, they had different diseases. They had different kinds of bone marrow transplants, with different outcomes. Their transplants were five years apart—a long time in bone marrow transplantation. In both instances, though, their transplants were attempts to save people who lacked, or could not use, the marrow of a conventionally matched donor. In this way, they both point to the future.

The type of transplant that saved Adam Schuler—a T-cell-depleted half-match—did not work for Patrick Thompson, who died in 1986 at fifteen, six years after he was diagnosed as having Hodgkin's disease, and several months after he had been found to have myelodysplasia as well. Neither his sisters nor his brother matched him at the critical HLA locus, and so he had three transplants from his parents—two from his father and one from his mother—during a hospitalization that lasted more than four months. It is not sure that any of the transplants engrafted at all, and it is certain that none engrafted for long.

Rappeport says nonengraftment is an instance for which he

would now use biological modifiers, developed since Patrick's death. These "colony-stimulating factors" are substances that, in some instances, enhance the ability of certain blood cells to proliferate. But this, too, would not necessarily—or even probably—have saved Patrick Thompson. Haploidentical transplants, though highly successful in SCID babies, do not work as well for older patients with other diseases, where both the existence of an immune system and the possibility of toxicity from the original problem may stymie new cells' efficacy. These factors, of course, are in addition to the difficulties inherent in overcoming a highly imperfect genetic match.

If Patrick were a patient today, says Rappeport, a full match from an unrelated donor would probably be his best option, but it was one that did not exist when he needed it. Of course there is no guarantee that—even if a donor could have been found—that would have worked either. But again progress is evident. It was possible to try, for Patrick, something that was unavailable only a short time earlier. And for a patient like him today, there would be more possibilities.

From the autopsy report on Patrick Thompson:

CLINICAL SUMMARY:

In March, 1980 this . . . white male presented with fever, malaise, cervical supraclavicular/axillary lymphadenopathy, and a large mediastinal mass. . . . Biopsy revealed *nodular sclerosing Hodgkin's disease*. . . . He received 6 courses of MOPP[1] chemotherapy. In 8/80 . . . he received 2400 rads to the mediastinum.

In 12/81 he had recurrence of night sweats. . . . Ultrasound revealed multiple masses around the liver. . . . He was empirically re-treated with MOPP.

In 2/82 he had disseminated Varicella, which was successfully treated with Varicel immunoglobulin, and ARA-C [almost certainly ARA-A, an antiviral drug]. In 3/82 he had a right middle lobe pneumonia, successfully treated with fluids and penicillin. By 7/82 6 additional courses of MOPP chemotherapy were completed. In 8/82 he was clinically asymptomatic, but some residual adenopathy was noted on CAT scans.

Between 9/82 and 4/83 he remained asymptomatic, but some growth of a right upper quadrant hypoechoic mass was noted. In 3/83 an exploratory laparotomy revealed retro-peritoneal lymphadenopathy. . . . Between 6/83 and 11/83 he received 6 cycles of "ABVD" combination chemotherapy. In 12/83 X-ray treatment of the splenipedicle and para-aortic nodes (2520 rads) was given.

Between 9/84 and 9/85 he became progressively pancytopenic, requiring intermittent RBC transfusions. A bone marrow aspirate showed . . . "dysplastic changes, ringed-sideroblasts and megalo-blastic changes." . . . Because of this "preleukemic" marrow, he was admitted to Brigham and Women's hospital on 8/27/85 for a bone marrow transplant from his haplo-identical father, with Leu-1 treatment. . . .

In other words, Patrick Thompson, after having been stricken with Hodgkin's disease when he was nine years old, underwent three courses of chemotherapy—each of which took place over a period of several months—and two of radiation. During the six-year period before he underwent a bone marrow transplant, he also suffered from pneumonia, and from a case of the chicken pox that nearly killed him; he received the varicella immunoglobulin, given to him in combination with an antiviral agent, on an emergency basis. Brian Smith says that people with Hodgkin's disease are immunodeficient—aside from or in addition to the effects of any chemotherapy they may be receiving—and virtually always get herpes zoster (chicken pox and/or shingles) if they've had chicken pox before. In addition to his illness and the sickness-inducing treatment for it, Patrick suffered through numerous painful and frightening tests. Eventually he developed myelodysplasia in addition to Hodgkin's disease, and by the summer before his transplant, he required regular blood transfusions.

Throughout, he remained a normal child, growing from a little boy to a six-foot-tall teenager. He was an altar boy. He had many, many friends. He played Little League ball, showing up for games the same day he had chemotherapy treatments. He'd go to the hospital early in the morning, come home and be sick, rest up, and be at the field in the early evening. On those days he played right field, but usually he pitched. "He was good, too," his father Rob says. His mother Nancy says she reminds Anne and Joe and Christina—Pat was the oldest of the four—that "Pat could be a real stinker sometimes," so that they will not unrealistically sanctify him, or feel inadequate to him as he is remembered. He was naive, but he had a certain wisdom, Rob and Nancy say. They are divorced now, and at the time they talked to me about Patrick had just separated. Though much pain showed, no acrimony did, and the story each of them told honored not only Patrick but each other. The sadness is in the washback.

As with all premature loss—that of the people I've portrayed and that which exists elsewhere—Patrick's death and its reverberations are heartbreaking, but his image and that of the family whose life he shared shine. I never saw Rob and Nancy Thompson together; they were living apart at the time of our interviews, and each spoke to me separately. But I have, in telling their story, intertwined their remarks, because in them they show themselves as united and agreed in their devotion to their son. They are as much Patrick's legacy as he would have been theirs, if life had gone as it should.

Rob is from Connecticut, where the Thompsons live now, and Nancy is from Cincinnati. They met in Michigan's Upper Peninsula, where they were both Vista Volunteers. After they were married, they moved to Hartford, and from there—while Rob was in the army—to Europe. Patrick was born in Italy. When Rob was discharged from the service, the family returned to Hartford, where Rob eventually joined the family insurance business. "My intention was never to be in this business, never to live in West Hartford. No way, José. But I realized I had an opportunity that was really remarkable. I was never pushed. I'm usually happy about the choice—it wasn't a gimme—and the job for me is very challenging." Anne and Joe were born, and—a couple of years after Patrick was diagnosed—Nancy had a miscarriage, and then Christina. Nancy went back to school, eventually majoring in theology.

Both Rob and Nancy, as they describe events with Patrick, show the life they had as the embodiment of good people's vision of happiness. They are tall and thin and athletic, lovers of the outdoors. References to camping trips taken and races run and flights of stairs climbed instead of bothering with the elevator illustrate their physical energy. Spiritual strength is also woven into their telling. Rob, a Catholic now, was a Congregationalist during Patrick's lifetime. Nancy has always been a Catholic. All the Thompsons are regular churchgoers. Rob and Nancy are both forthright, forceful, and unaffected about the peace and grace God and prayer give them and about the help the institutional Church and its representatives—priests and nuns—has been. They are grateful members of their community, and it is plain they are giving ones as well. In their bearing, in their tone, and in their language they show an active reflectiveness: They thought before they spoke with Patrick or made decisions about him, and they do the same in their lives now. Though they are sure of their standards and values, they continually examine their application.

The Thompsons are not perfect. They have problems, between themselves and no doubt within themselves. But they have an ethos—of thoughtfulness, of social action, of appreciation, of effort—that seems the maturation of the best of 1960s liberalism, of American energy and generosity, and this suffuses their experience.

First, there was the diagnosis, "in the fall of the year Patrick was nine," Nancy says, "whatever year that was. It must have been in 1980—1979 to 1980—when he was in the third grade. He had had his regular school checkup, and everything was fine. Then around Christmastime everybody got the flu bug. And Pat never seemed to recover. After dinner he would go and lie down on the couch and fall asleep. It was unbelievably out of character for him. He was like Ready Kilowatt, always tearing around, and full of energy. Plus, he woke up with night sweats. Several times. In the morning he'd wake up, and his pajama top would be damp. I was so naive and had absolutely no knowledge about symptoms for cancer. For Hodgkin's. So it didn't really scare me; I thought it was part of his cold or his flu or whatever."

In fact, according to Brian Smith, the mechanism behind the night sweats associated with Hodgkin's disease isn't all that different from that behind a reaction to cold and flu viruses. "Presumably it is magic mediators. These things that cells ordinarily make—cytokines—make various things to control other cells. Some of the things they make change your blood vessel contractility, to make you sweat and do all those kinds of things. That's what happens when you get a cold and you get a fever. It isn't so much the virus that gives you that—it's actually your body reacting against the virus that gives you the fever, and gives you the sweats, and gives you all of that stuff. And that's why people who take interferon, for example, and those kinds of things, feel like they have the flu sometimes. Cytokines are the thing that makes you do it. I don't know why it's at night, with Hodgkin's. That nobody knows."

Patrick went to the doctor, "I think on a Saturday morning," says Nancy. "We were supposed to go pick up a new camper that day. A pop-up Coleman camper. I was getting the other kids ready and everything. So Rob took him to the doctor."

The doctor found a lump under Patrick's arm. Later, the little boy said he'd known it was there; he'd thought it was a muscle.

"My memory is that the doctor wanted to rule some things

out," Rob says, "and get this chest X ray. I don't remember being overly concerned at the time. My memory is that I wasn't really alarmed. I took him over to the radiologists, and they did the chest X ray, and it showed this massive—this mass in his chest." The tumor had metastasized. "And Pat was immediately in the hospital as of that day. That afternoon. They didn't give a name to it then, because they didn't know what the name was. We assumed—I guess thought it was a cancerous something. And my memory of that is it was pretty traumatic for everybody. And that's when it started."

"They removed the lump," Nancy says. "And they sent it to pathology, and it was a long week of waiting. Well, I don't know if it was a week; it seemed like forever. I can't remember exactly how long it was. It was a couple of days. They did the whole battery of tests. I can't remember everything they did. But it seemed like every day there was something else scheduled."

Right from the start, the Thompsons established their modus operandi with Patrick. All medical information was to go through them to Patrick. They, not the doctors, would decide what their child was to know about his illness. They assured him the most normal life possible by protecting him from fear, following their instincts and using their good sense. They told him he had Hodgkin's disease, but they did not use the word "cancer." Nancy Thompson has a calm, sweet voice, very quiet when she talks about the pain her child suffered, but clear the rest of the time. Rob's has a hearty sound. He retraces sad history, sometimes while crying, with all the objectivity he can muster. The phrase "My memory is" recurs frequently in his scrupulous account. The impression the Thompsons make is overwhelmingly one of reasonableness. They prevailed.

During one of the tests on Patrick, "The doctor said I could not stay," Nancy says, "and I absolutely would not leave. And he said, 'You have to leave.' And I said, 'I promised this kid that I wouldn't leave him.' And Pat was on the table, and he was terrified. I said, 'You have to let me stay at least until you get those needles in.' He said, 'I'm sorry, Mrs. Thompson, you can't stay,' and he went in to wash his hands. Well, I turned around and went right after him, right into where he was washing his hands. And I said, 'Look, I'm going to withdraw consent if you don't allow me to stay.' And we got into it. And finally I guess he threw his hands up and said, 'I've never done this before' [allowed a parent to be present], and I said, 'Well, I haven't either. And neither has my son.' So he allowed me to stay for ten or fifteen minutes."

For the next few years, Patrick's life was "amazingly—I'm not going to say *normal*," Rob says, "but he didn't miss a heck of a lot. Pat was just—he was a loving kid. He was a sensitive boy. But he wasn't a goody two-shoes. He was sharp as a tack, but he was innocent in so many ways. You know, the altar boy innocence. For instance, when he graduated from the eighth grade, he was given the good citizenship award."

All this during round after round of chemotherapy. "I don't remember the regimen myself," Rob says. "But there were the pills, and there were the injections and the bone marrow tests and the whole megillah, and you had to psych yourself and him up for them. That was a bugger. That was just rough."

Up until the time of the transplant, "He didn't lose his hair. Got thin at times, but he never became bald. He was prepared—well, I don't know if he was prepared for it, but we talked about it a lot—but he never had to deal with that with his peers, which was a real blessing." Both the Thompsons were constantly frightened that someone would scare Patrick with the threatening possibilities of his disease, the very aspects of it they were withholding. There was only one such incident, after Patrick had his spleen taken out, and a child on the school bus told him she'd known someone who'd had the same thing done and had died.

Patrick's face "would balloon up," Rob says, from the steroids that were part of his regimen, but generally he looked fine, and that normalcy helped insulate him from the terror his parents were bent on keeping from him. If his hair had fallen out, Rob says, "that could have been a real toughie."

Throughout—in fact, up to days before Patrick died—the Thompsons maintained optimism. Although, "It was not uncommon for me," says Rob, "when Pat was living—when I was running—for me to think about the fact that Pat might not live. A run is a private time, a reflective time. I used to run in a park called Woodland Park, and I can even right this minute picture myself in a certain spot, thinking about that. And another specific spot, a treed area, along a golf course. I remember thinking about the fact that Pat could die."

And Nancy says, "I can remember when Pat was initially diagnosed. The surgeon relayed it to the pediatrician, and the pediatrician called Rob at work. And apologized for not being able to talk to him in person. And I can remember Rob calling me, and telling me that Pat had Hodgkin's disease, and I can still see myself standing in the dining room window talking on the phone, and when I got off the phone something—intuition, or just a gut feeling—I just *knew* that eventually he was going to die from this. I didn't want to believe it, and I pushed it out of my mind, but I had this overwhelming feeling that he would die from it."

This is despite the fact that when a name was put to Patrick's disease, the Thompsons were relieved to hear it wasn't worse. "You know," says Rob, "to be happy with a diagnosis of Hodgkin's disease was true. As opposed to—what we feared. Rampant leukemia and stuff like that." The cure rate for Hodgkin's disease is over 70 percent, with younger people and those whose cases are diagnosed earlier doing better than the others. Some of the tests Patrick had when he was first diagnosed were to determine the extent of his disease; the process is called "staging," and the results are categorized from I to IV (I being the most limited and IV the most pervasive) and as either A, indicating the patient is asymptomatic, or B, that he or she suffers from significant weight loss, spiking fever, or night sweats. Patrick was stage III B, the III being defined as "involvement of lymph node regions on both sides of the diaphragm, which may include localized involvement of an extra-lymphatic site . . . or spleen. . . or both."[2]

Patrick was tested regularly for the recurrence of disease. It seemed to Nancy that it was always Christmastime when some kind of testing had to be done. "And it was always holding your breath. I can remember on Christmas Eve, in fact, they did a test. And the test was negative, so that was our Christmas present." But Patrick did relapse, with Hodgkin's twice, and then, starting in 1984, he developed myelodysplasia. (Roberta's illness took much the same course, except that when she was first diagnosed it was with more advanced Hodgkin's disease—stage IV.)

"Whenever he relapsed," Nancy says, "it was devastating. We knew that Hodgkin's was one of the best cancers to have if you had to have cancer, if it's possible to say such a thing. And the cure rate was much better. And that if you got past five years, or seven years, you could almost be considered a cure. So it was just devastating.

"And even though, in the beginning, he was wonderful about his treatments, as the years progressed, I can remember that two or three days before he would start his therapy, the whole family would react, anticipating what was coming up. Probably starting on Monday or Tuesday. He would always have the treatment on Friday. That would give him the weekend to recover, so he only had to miss one day of school. By Thursday he was pretty down. Got real quiet and sullen.

"After I had the miscarriage—or before I did—we got into the routine of Rob taking him for his treatments and then bringing him home and I would care for him the rest of the day. And what would happen is he would get sick in the afternoon—start in the afternoon—and then he'd sleep and I'd try to give him the Compazine to settle his stomach so he could sleep even more. And usually by nine or ten o'clock at night he'd be feeling a little bit better, and he'd come down and have a bite to eat and then he'd go back upstairs." He vomited, Nancy says. "Lots. So the other kids would just be really quiet. They knew that was his sick day.

"Pat was a real easy kid. He was agreeable. He could protest, but when he knew he had to do something, he'd put up a fight and then, 'All right, let's do it.' That was with regard to everything. But one morning, we couldn't find him. And the poor little thing was down the basement. Hiding. 'Cause he didn't want to go for his treatment. Because he was just . . . It seems to me that toward the last year it was just extremely hard on him."

In May of 1985 a bone marrow aspiration confirmed myelodysplasia, and the Thompsons started talking about options "that weren't that great." None, other than a bone marrow transplant, "that we felt were reliable," says Nancy. "You know, vitamin therapy." Patrick's Hartford doctor referred the Thompsons to the Brigham. The first time, Nancy and Rob went alone, without Patrick.

"We had all of Patrick's medical records," Nancy says. "Rob had made a couple of trips to Boston with medical records. Scans and stuff like that. 'Cause when they wanted them, they wanted them. Right away. And we didn't want to trust them to the mails."

When it comes to medical care, Rob says, "You have to be your own quarterback, because nobody else is doing it. You know, you have this perception that there's somebody back here kind of fielding the whole deal and keeping an eye on everything, and coordinating all the efforts and all this stuff. You may think there is, but there isn't. You have to follow through and pursue things and do some coordination and follow-up and all those things. Just as you do in *anything*—so it's true in the medical area. Whether it's a very difficult thing or not. If more doctors get involved, it requires more coordination.

"Doctors are not necessarily business people. They don't always have the same follow-through techniques and so forth that business people have to make sure everybody's getting the same information and knows what's going on and who's doing what. People in business are more apt to be involved in overall planning, and certainly planning's involved when you're dealing with the follow-through on a problem like Pat had. But there are so many doctors that get interjected into the flow of things, it takes someone like a parent to make sure this doctor"—Rob slaps his desk—"knows what that doctor"—another slap—"said. Because it might be very important that a doctor have the information the next time he goes around and not three weeks later, when he gets a memo. The file might look good, and their rear end'll be covered, but the patient might be dead by then."

Rob had hoped Patrick could be maintained indefinitely on transfusions. "He'd get tanked up by a transfusion, and it would be like a shot of Adrenalin. Amazing. And then he'd just start to slow down. You would think that he could be transfused for the rest of his life, but that doesn't happen. We were told that sooner or later it's not going to work. Or he's probably going to develop— something's going to happen. And that the only chance that Pat really had for long life was a bone marrow transplant.

"We went up and talked with Brian. What a wonderful guy. Just—he's got a way—is such a gentle man. He told us about the procedure. Ultimately, we knew that when we were dealing with a half-match situation, the odds were really stinko. I don't know if he said 20–25 percent or maybe in that neck of the woods."

Smith's chief recollection of the meeting is of his surprise that the Thompsons had not told Patrick that he had cancer and his insistence that they do so. "I remember we were having this perfectly logical transplant conversation. You know, it was haplo," a genetic half-match between donor and recipient. "Nobody did this. So we went over graft-versus-host disease and T-cell depletion and his disease, and the variety of other criteria for a transplant, like how his liver was and how his lungs were and all these other things that might preclude him from being a candidate. Then we had this twenty-minute discussion about how—you know—we didn't do transplants as a mystery."

"We started to use the word 'cancer' with him," Rob says,

"when we went up to Boston, or maybe when we were at Boston. I can't remember when, exactly. I remember we had to deal with the word 'leukemia' with him. That was traumatic. That was hard. And how he had a preleukemic condition."

"Pat knew he had Hodgkin's disease," Nancy says, "and that it was a disease of his blood. And I don't think we ever talked about—we didn't really discuss cancer with him. We did when we were in Boston for the transplant. I think we were all pretty frightened."

During Nancy and Rob's first visit to Boston, Smith told them the hard facts. "All the kids had been tested, and we had been tested, for HLA matching," Nancy says. "And the other children were not compatible. So we discussed that. And what the chances were. And the percentages. And that was pretty frightening—it was very frightening. It was awful. Probably one of the worst days of my life. Ever. Getting that news. Wanting him to say, '*But,* this is what we can do. This looks awful, and these things are awful, but this is what we're going to do, and everything's going to be all right.' And of course he never said that.

"Brian just has this wonderful manner about him and was very kind and careful about how he talked to us and told us things. But I can remember the first time I ever met Joel Rappeport. Here's this guy come buzzing down the hall and buzzing back up, and he was just so busy and everything. Brian pulled him in [to the examining room where they were talking] and said, 'I want you to meet the Thompsons.'

"He came in and he had this big smile on his face," Nancy says, "and he was laughing about something that had happened, or he was telling Brian something, and all I can remember is thinking, 'My God, why is this man smiling?' My whole world— I had just been told in so many words that my son was going to die, unless a miracle happened. And he was smiling. The rest of the world was smiling, too. It wasn't just him.

"I can remember coming back on the Mass Pike and finally Rob just pulled over and we sat in one of the rest stops and the two of us just cried. Just held each other and cried. For the longest time."

At home, they told Patrick. Rob says, "I remember distinctly telling Pat—and it was telling Pat, it wasn't asking Pat—telling Pat that we were going to Boston to do this."

"We explained to him that he was going to get a bone marrow

transplant," Nancy says. "Patrick said, 'This sounds pretty serious, Dad. Could I die from this? Am I going to die?' And I believe Rob said, 'No, everything's going to be okay.'

"I said, 'No,' " Rob says, "I told him, 'No.' " Rob says it as if it were a promise, one he still appears to be glad he made.

"Then when Rob explained he was going to be the donor, and sort of explained in a very elementary way how they did a bone marrow transplant, Pat started to cry," Nancy says. "And we said, 'Why are you crying, exactly?' and he said to Rob, 'Because then you won't have any bone marrow.' "

"His response," Rob says, crying, "was one of concern for me."

Other than that, Patrick's concerns were about his normal life, particularly about starting high school—Northwest Catholic—with his friends. Rob and Nancy said Patrick would be going into the hospital about that time, but that they would look into tutoring and hoped that when he got back, he would be able to pick up where he left off. Then Rob took Patrick and a friend golfing.

That summer, Nancy says, anticipating that Patrick was going into the hospital and what the outcome might be, they did a lot. "We went to Rob's college reunion, in Maine. We took the whole family and went to Disney World for a week. In early August everybody flew to Chicago to my brother's wedding. And my whole family was there. That was pretty much the last time a lot of them saw Patrick. Then, in the week before we went to Boston, we took another week and rented a condo up in the White Mountains and had a nice time up there, and came back on a Sunday or a Monday, and the next day or two—Tuesday or Wednesday—we took him to Boston."

Patrick Thompson was admitted to the Brigham and Women's Hospital the end of August 1985 and died there January 5, 1986. At first, Nancy and Rob both stayed in Boston, and then, after a few weeks, took turns, with Nancy spending the week there and Rob coming on weekends, when—usually—Nancy returned to the rest of the family. First Rob's parents and then Nancy's took care of Annie and Joey and Chrissie, who came often to visit their brother. The nearby Boston Ronald McDonald House, like the one in New Haven, is beautifully decorated and equipped and was a great boon. At a cost of ten dollars a day the Thompsons, Nancy especially, lived there for much of the time Patrick was hospitalized. Sometimes Nancy and Rob had dinner together Friday nights, but often,

Rob says, they would just see each other's car as they passed on the turnpike going in opposite directions. Hartford is about ninety miles from Boston.

"My first meeting with Joel Rappeport scared the living tar out of me," Rob Thompson says. He is referring to their first long talk, not to the initial greeting in the examining room. "My gut feeling was, Here's this big-timer from Boston with this— approach, which is very different from Brian's. My memory of Brian is very gentle, soft-spoken, sensitive, considerate—and yet informative. And not assuming a lot. The initial impression Joel made on me was almost the opposite of all those things. Big-city-hospital brusqueness and get-with-the-program-here-buddy and this-is-the-way-we-do-it-here kind of thing. That got changed as I saw the softer, loving side of him. And as he saw and came to know Pat, he changed. No question in my mind about that. I think he came to know Pat pretty well. He is indeed a sensitive, loving man. And brighter than most people all put together. But he's not a real smoothie. Doesn't have to be.

"I remember having to tell Joel exactly what Pat's perception of everything was, that this might be a real advanced teaching hospital and all that stuff, but we're dealing with a fourteen-year-old boy here. You don't have to tell him that if this doesn't work, he may die. That's not what you're going to tell him. He said, 'Well, this is the way we do it.' And I said, 'Well, that's not the way you're doing it with Patrick.' He bought it. He didn't have any choice. I guess he could have said, 'Okay, you're leaving.' Then I don't know what we'd have done. But he had to meet Pat, he had to get to know Pat. It's not a piece of meat there. I don't think he thought that it was, but it was another patient. I got to appreciate Joel much more as time went on. Tremendously. Indeed, love him. But I didn't at first. My memory of that first visit was just that he was going to tell all, that we were going to be up-front about everything, and we said, 'We're not going to tell him any lies, but we're not going to maybe tell him all.' That's the importance of family being around a patient. They need an advocate. Younger people do, for sure. So that worked itself out, but we were always on the defense. I can almost feel defensive right now, put myself back in that position. Glad I'm not doing that anymore."

The first transplant, from Rob, was September 12, 1985. Like the marrow administered to Jennie Gossom, Rob's was treated with Anti-leu 1. This was necessary to try to avert the horrendous GVH that would otherwise, in this instance, be a virtual certainty, although, Rappeport says, any such manipulation of the marrow reduces its volume by half.

"The damnedest thing happened," Rob says. "In part of this spinning-down process, or whatever the process is, they lost some of the marrow. Because the bag broke. They told us. They said the amount that was given was reduced. But it was just an outright goof. It was a hell of a thing. It was just unbelievable."

"I couldn't believe it," Nancy says. "I'll never forget when they told me that. Rob was lying in the room, groggy. And Joel came in and Brian and somebody else—a whole tribe came in. I'm not sure if this was before or after they gave Pat the marrow. Probably before. But they told me that, and I went crazy. It was like, Here was *the* chance to save my son's life and you broke the bag? At that point I was not a person who swore. But I think I said, 'Goddammit! Jesus!' I don't know what I said. Something like that. I wasn't swearing at anybody. It was just—I was in shock. How could this happen? It never crossed my mind that something like that could happen."

Neither Rappeport nor Smith told me about the bag breaking—I heard about it from the Thompsons—but when I asked them if it had affected the outcome for Patrick, neither seemed surprised by my question and each answered me fully. Rappeport said simply that he didn't know. "That is just unanswerable," he said, and the sadness in his tone was the most convincingly caring statement anyone could make.

Smith said, too, "We'll never know." But he doesn't think it made a difference. "If the problem was that he didn't get enough stem cells with the first graft, then there's two things. One is what you'd expect to happen—that he would take a long time to come in." As with Adam Schuler. The fact that Jennie Gossom, also with myelodysplasia and T-cell-depleted marrow, quickly regenerated simply shows how many factors are not known, what's left to be learned, because neither Rappeport nor Smith has an explanation for the difference.

Smith, continuing about Patrick says, "It would take a very long time for the graft to come in, and it might even cycle. Because it turns out that the number of emerging stem cells, and more especially their progeny—granulocytes, platelets, etc.—do go up and down in quantity quite a lot. So it would just take a very, very long time. What he did was much more classic graft rejection, like you see in aplastic anemia sometimes: Things come and then, plunk! They crash. And if you look at Patrick Thompson's blood, he had residual cells of his own, capable of killing off the donor. You're never going to know for absolutely sure, but it makes you think that the mechanism was to mount an active immune response against those stem cells. Maybe if you could get 10 to 100 times the number of stem cells, you could eventually overwhelm them. But a third more, a half more, twice as many stem cells—just doesn't overwhelm them. I mean, the stem cells are just too potent. So it really seemed to be an immunological rejection. We try to distinguish rejection from failure. The other thing is, if it was just a matter of enough stem cells, you'd expect the second and the third transplants to work."

On October 15, Patrick received a second transplant, again from Rob. "The first time," Rappeport says, "he had been prepared with ARA-C, Cytoxan,[3] and total body irradiation. Plus, we added in the drug VP 16. For the second, we were more concerned about nonengraftment, and we treated it as if it were aplastic anemia. Because he didn't engraft, didn't have any bone marrow left, and now you're not trying to get rid of malignant cells. So he got Cytoxan, ATS, procarbazine, and cyclosporine. And before the third one, because he'd gotten all this, and we didn't think he could get much more, he just got antithymocyte serum." The long list of toxic agents boggles the mind, but it was not all that was going on. There were the usual antibiotics and antiemetics and, in Patrick's case, even more. When his Hickman catheter was implanted, a mass was found in his chest, and so, the autopsy report says, "during the transplant protocol he was also receiving X-ray therapy for his Hodgkin's disease."

Patrick's father was the donor for the first two transplants because, says Smith, "we did the father on the old pregnancy issue; when a woman is pregnant, she can become sensitized to her child, once outside pregnancy. In marrow transplantation that means Nancy's marrow was—theoretically—more likely to induce GVH in Patrick than Rob's was. There was no evidence of that, but we figure if we're going to flip a coin— We didn't know enough not to do it that way at the time."

"We'd still do it that way," Rappeport says.

After the transplant from Nancy, there was apparent reason for hope: nucleated red cells appeared. But they are really not the certain harbinger of good news that they're held out to be, according to Rappeport. "Although it's a measure of some function of bone marrow, we use it as an indicator that the patient has had engraftment, and that is probably not strictly true. After all, one has just put in this free-floating bone marrow, and in fact just from the maturation process there could be a nucleated red or so. On the other hand, if one sees it there a week or more later, it's not something that would have just matured up from what one put in but should represent some sort of growth phenomenon. I don't think nucleated red cells appearing after a week represent engraftment for the following reason, though: It's the pluripotent stem cell that we're interested in, and given what little is known about the kinetics of it, it is conceivable that it is really weeks to months later before that cell actually comes all the way through. That's probably engraftment [the appearance of stem cells], and I don't think we have a measure of it, and we don't use it—because we don't have any way to do that. But I think someday that will be what we use to measure engraftment, rather than maturation of a moderately mature cell."

Day after day, during over four months of hospitalization, the Thompsons waited for Patrick's blood counts to come up.

"What I remember mostly," Brian Smith says "is going there" to Patrick's room "and having to have this there-are-no-blood-counts discussion every day." The Thompsons responded to that, he says, "patiently and with concern. I don't know what 'appropriate' means, but . . ."

"Rather than 'appropriate,' " Rappeport says of the Thompsons, echoing his disavowal of the phrase "out of line" when trying to describe Reba Folsom's educated and involved questions, "I would say they were with us. Wanted to know the facts, wanted to know what our opinions were, but they were just basically with us in both concern and understanding."

"We were just totally positive—upbeat—about the whole deal," Rob says. "Up to hours before he died. I mean, I look back on that now, and I say that was an illusion. But that's okay. I don't say, 'You dummy,' you know. We take care of ourselves in our own way. And thank goodness. You find hope in lots of little things; you find something to grab on to."

"The Christmas that we had up there," Nancy says, "was the most beautiful, the most meaningful Christmas we ever had as a family." Nancy's parents came, and from the twenty-third on, Anne and Joe and Christina were there, as well as Rob and Nancy.

"Patrick had a faith in God, he believed in God," says Nancy. "He was raised a Catholic and went to parochial schools all his life. But he was a typical kid, he didn't like to go to church. When he was in the hospital, he didn't want to have the Anointing of the Sick—what they used to call the Last Rites. Patrick hadn't wanted to have anything to do with it. Then before I gave the marrow, I wanted to have the Anointing of the Sick. I said to Pat, 'Look, I'm going to be anointed, you want to do it too? We'll do it together.' He said okay, so we had a big ceremony up on the floor, and the priest and I sort of planned it together. He anointed us, and we had communion, and we invited some of the staff that we were close to. And then, right before Christmas—I think it was the twenty-third—we—I—wanted to have a communion service for Pat. And the priest said, 'Oh, no, we can't do that. We've never done that before.' I said, 'Look, I really think it's important. These people— He's totally isolated. The one thing he doesn't have is a church service, or spirituality. It's so void up here, it's so antiseptic.' He said, 'What if other people find out about it?' I said, 'What if they did! Wouldn't that be wonderful!' So he said okay, but it won't be a real Mass. It won't be this, it won't be that. I said okay.

"And I can remember at the end of the communion service, I was supposed to do the last prayer, and I stepped into the doorway of the flow room, and the priest was there, and I was all ready to begin to read this prayer, and all the adults were ready to get on with it. I started to read, and then I looked up and Pat was still—he had received communion, and he still had his head bowed, and his hands folded and his eyes closed, and he was still praying. So we waited, and when he was finished, he looked up and kind of smiled, and we proceeded on. That was real special.

"Rob and I spent Christmas Eve with Patrick, in the unit. The nurses had a buffet in the nurses' station, and we brought something for that—we were part of that—and Joel was there. My mom and dad and Annie and I went to midnight Mass, and on Christmas morning, really early, around six or seven, Rob went over and saw Pat."

"We really planned that Christmas," Rob says. "Pat wrapped presents, and we had presents sterilized, and some were in the room, and some were out of the room. He never had so many damn presents." He gave them, too—choosing them from catalogues a social worker (Martha Burke, who then did Patrick's Christmas shopping) had sterilized and brought to him—not only to his family but to the nurses and doctors and other hospital workers who were by then his friends. Patrick gave a pair of argyle socks to a favorite doctor—Gary Gilliland, who later took care of Roberta—and a pen to his father and a stuffed animal, a white Christmas goose, to his little sister. "We got pooped wrapping and unwrapping," Rob says.

"Pat had all his presents," Nancy says. "It took him about three hours. He sat up on his bed and opened them—those that weren't sterilized he opened through the plastic. And he was exhausted, but he had a ball. We spread blankets on the floor, and the kids opened their presents, and the staff were all part of it. That was a really beautiful day for us."

"But then," Rob says, "everything went downhill from there. I had to go back to Connecticut, and Nancy stayed on. And things started to happen. Complications. Lung problems. What finally happened is I got a telephone call from Nance on a Friday night, and she said, 'Rob, I think you better get up here. Pat's having a very difficult time and—you better get here as soon as you can.'

"I got there sometime after midnight. I will never forget the scene I walked into. I would like to rid my mind of that thought. You know the laminar flow rooms and the cleanliness routine and the whole bit? You have the open door, and you have the wall through which you have the gloves and so forth. Well, that whole thing moves. And that whole wall was open. Everything had gone to the wind. All I can picture is just—people. All around there. And a lot of white coats. And Pat. And what they were doing was—they were intubating Pat.

"Oh, God, it was just so dreadful. He was fighting that. But they had to. I mean, he just wasn't getting enough oxygen. But Pat had seen those machines. He knew that the fellow who was in the room before him had had them, and he knew that that guy had died. He had voiced this with Nance beforehand. And they had talked—that he had to do this. That for Pat it was just another thing he had to do. And then he would come out the other side and that he would get back to business. That's the way he accepted it. But the actual physical part of it was— You know, I hate those machines. It's done wonderful things.[4] But it didn't in our case.

"Nancy and I set up shop in a room down the hall. And he died about a day later. I was taking a nap, and Nance was over at the McDonald House changing, and a nurse came charging in, woke me up and said, 'Mr. Thompson, come quickly, Pat's blood pressure is declining rapidly.' He was not awake then. But you know what was so wonderful? That we could hug him and kiss him and hold him."

"All the nurses," Nancy says, "the primary nurses—all came back within an hour after Pat died, and helped pack up all of his stuff. I guess they had all known that he was going to die. And they had left word that when he died, they wanted to be notified, and they all came in, and they packed up all of his stuff, and that was on Sunday morning. And they all came to the funeral."

The day Patrick died, "I stayed over," Nancy says. "Rob wanted me to come home that Sunday night. I said, 'I can't, I have to wait and bring Patrick home.' Because I felt that I just couldn't leave at that point. I guess I just wasn't accepting. Rob had called the funeral director, a man who was a member of our church, and made the arrangements."

On Monday, Nancy waited at the front of the hospital with Martha Burke, the social worker who was by now a dear friend, for the hearse. "And I told Randy [the funeral director] to follow me, because I was going to lead the way home. 'Cause I didn't think I could bear to follow him." And on the spur of the moment she decided to drive over to the Ronald McDonald House with the hearse following, because Pat had always thought he would see it sometime. "He was always asking about the house and what it was like, and if he would have to wear a mask, and all that," Nancy says. "So when we left the hospital, we drove over to the house, and Randy had no idea where we were going. I didn't tell him, I just did it, and then we turned around. Instead of going the short way to the Mass Pike, we went past Fenway Park, and then we got on the Mass Pike and came home.

"And when we came home, I told Randy that I wanted to go past our house. So we came past the house one more time. That was not something that I had planned, either. It was just something that happened. And I'm glad. It made me feel better."

Dear Dr. Rappeport,

Thank you for your letter and your very kind words about Patrick. I have to agree with you that Patrick was indeed a very special young man. I am so proud to be his mother.

Thank you for the excellent care that you and all of the doctors and staff . . . gave to Patrick and to Rob and me. I think your entire staff—the doctors, the nurses, the support people—are all very special people who care a great deal about all of the patients and give them the best possible medical and personal care. We are extremely grateful that we had the opportunity to bring our son to you, and we have no regrets.

As you said, despite that fact that Patrick died, something very positive and good did come out of the whole experience.

We would like to meet with you and discuss the final autopsy report. Please just let us know when you have it, and we can decide on a date that would be convenient for all of us.

We certainly don't plan to lose touch with all of the new friends we made in Boston and particularly at the Brigham. So please let us know if there is any way we can help you. We are especially interested in the progress of the new adult recovery house and hope you won't hesitate to call on us if there is anything at all we can do to help you out. I sincerely mean it.

Thank you again for all that you did for us. Take care.

Sincerely,
Nancy N. Thompson

From the autopsy report on Patrick Thompson:

Pre-terminally, on about 1/1–1/5/86 he developed progressive respiratory distress . . . a pericardial catheter was placed, and 800 cc of straw-colored fluid was drained. He was emergently intubated on 1/3/85 . . . By the evening of 1/3/85 [actually 1/3/86], the chest X ray was "total white-out." He expired at 9:30 AM on 1/5/86.

Autopsy Summary and Discussion:
Respiratory failure was due to a bilaterally severe interstitial pneumonitis, with superimposed hyaline membrane formation. The cause of this process is unknown. . . .

Interstitial pneumonitis is a recognized complication of bone marrow transplantation. . . . It is yet unclear what role chemotherapeutic agents, radiation, immune reactions, or occult viral infections play in causing this disease. . . .

Residual Hodgkin's disease was not found at autopsy. . . . The bone marrow contained scattered small foci of immature, but normally differentiating, myeloid and erythroid cells. Megakaryocytes were notably absent. It therefore appears that the intended purpose of the bone marrow transplant may have been partly successful.

"I'll never know the suffering that he went through," Nancy says now. "Some people I've talked to who've had a transplant have said, 'I'd never do it again. I'd rather die.' And so I wonder if he felt that way. I guess the only thing that haunts me at times is if I should have been more honest—more truthful—about the seriousness of it. Of his chances. Even with a child, does a parent have the right to withhold that information? That worries me. Should I have been more open and forthright? Were we denying what was going on? I don't think that we were. I think the way we handled Patrick, the way we handled the situation, was very—right on, with him. I guess one of the things that got Pat through was that he trusted us. And believed what we said. I believed that he would make it."

"To communicate a lot of negative stuff," Rob says, "just wasn't fitting. I wouldn't say that I would do it differently. Knowing Pat, my answer still comes up: No, I wouldn't have done it differently. We dealt with Pat in regard to the disease in the same way that perhaps you might answer a youngster asking about sex: We answered his questions but didn't read into them. We answered them very literally, as best we could. And answered them to the degree that Pat wanted to hear the answers."

"We'll never know how difficult it was for him," Nancy says. "Being young. And really what his thoughts were. I think he tried to protect us as much as we tried to protect him. Basically, though, I think he thought he was going to get better. I don't think he thought he was going to die, although that did cross his mind. I think he trusted us.

"I like to think that as much as he was in pain, and with all the agony of what the radiation and the chemotherapy do to someone, if he hadn't had the transplant—if he had stayed home and just been transfused—that it would have been a very long and hard death for Pat. He may have died sooner, but he certainly would've been much more aware of what was happening. And at least the way it worked out, he had hope. We all did. We all had hope."

The Reverend Jane Morse, an Episcopal priest, did have an absolutely exact donor—herself. She had an autologous transplant—one in which the patient's own marrow is harvested and then, after he or she has received further treatment, reinfused. As Rappeport says, the word "transplant" is inaccurate in this instance, because an organ is not being moved from one person to another. Nevertheless, the procedure for an autologous transplant is much the same as for an allogeneic (from person to person) or syngeneic one (specifically between identical twins), and the object is the same: to cure the patient of disease. Furthermore, autologous transplants, like haploidentical ones, hold out great hope for the many people without a conventional donor.

So far—over the two years since Jane's transplant for recurrent non-Hodgkin's lymphoma—the effort seems to have been a success. She is well, back to her usual life with her husband and young adult daughter and son, and anxious about finishing work for a Ph.D. at Yale Divinity School. Though Rappeport is skeptical about the widespread applicability of autologous transplants, he thinks that at her age (forty-six at the time of transplant) and for her disease (one that does not affect the stem cell) it is the best choice.

"In the future," says Rappeport, "I think autologous transplantation will be used more for the following reasons, none of which are good scientific reasons: It's easier; you don't have to understand anything about transplantation to do it."

He stands up, closes the door of the conference room in which we're meeting so he can have a secret cigarette—the building has a prohibition against smoking—gets himself a paper cup of coffee and a doughnut, and sits down again. He is in a terrible mood, chiefly because an old patient's new doctor has not consulted with him over her current treatment. Rappeport found this out after talking to the patient's husband, and now he's both furious and depressed, feeling excluded from continuing and developing therapy he instigated for her many years ago, and frustrated at not being able to participate in her care; he's sure he understands her complex symptoms better than anyone else does and could help her more.

"You might not even have to do it, and you could do it and get away with it," he says, ostensibly speaking about autologous transplants, but with an unarticulated subtext about all ill-considered, badly defined treatment. "So I think it's going to be extraordinarily popular. Do I think it is justified? No. It's easier to set up a program [for autologous rather than allogeneic transplants], and programs are set up not necessarily with the patient in mind. But it's a way to say you offer a bone marrow transplant program, so that you can tell the community that you're doing this, so that you can have patients sent to you, so you can generate more money and a bigger clinic, so you can attract trainees, or continue to attract trainees.

"I'm not against autologous totally. I just think it gets misused. And I'm against its misuse. I think we all may be misusing it. I think in fact patients may not need transplants for these lymphomas. They may just need the chemotherapy and good production [of blood cells]. I think the chemotherapy mavens need to figure out whether one needs to use bone marrow transplant in lymphomas. In this situation," if the marrow was not destroyed but its function profoundly suppressed, "the use of a growth factor might replace autologous transplantation." It is the objective scientist talking. "But I think to take an isolated patient and not give the marrow back," says Rappeport, the personally involved clinician, "one would have some difficulty doing that." The effectiveness of a patient's chemotherapy isn't known for a long time, he says, and so "taking the bone marrow and giving it back to her is probably a relatively benign process."

"I think the justifications for doing autologous transplantation are very clear. And they are that you have a disease for which you have an effective treatment, but said treatment is limited by virtue of irreversible toxicity to the bone marrow. Very simple. You know, it's been tried in virtually every solid tumor." He doesn't believe it works in any of them, however, with the exception of "a small group of testicular cancers, and Ewing's sarcoma," a cancer of the bone. "In people who have relapsed."

I ask him about the child he transplanted who had retinoblastoma, the rare eye cancer that afflicts children. "He's doing okay," Rappeport says, but no informative sample exists; only three children in the world have been treated this way. Autologous transplants as adjunct therapy for people with solid tumors "may have a role. A drug may come out tomorrow that has tremendous efficacy against—pick a tumor—but which is truly limited by its toxicity to bone marrow. Irreversible toxicity to bone marrow. Then autologous transplantation becomes a very viable option. It's just that the criteria are not being fulfilled."

Several months after this conversation, Rappeport had another one, with a representative of Blue Cross/Blue Shield, on the advisability of health insurance providers paying for bone marrow transplants administered to patients with breast cancer so that they can survive otherwise lethal chemotherapy. He's still in doubt about whether the procedure will work, but his advice is to pay for it, because, he says, that will be a way to find out if it's a viable therapy. Blue Cross/Blue Shield, under considerable public pressure, does decide to pay for bone marrow transplants for breast cancer, and Rappeport's pleased with whatever part he may have played in forming policy. The insurance company, by footing the bill, will in effect be financing clinical research and thus helping to find the truth.

"There are a few diseases in which autologous transplantation is probably of some value," Rappeport says. "Hodgkin's disease, non-Hodgkin's lymphoma, and neuroblastoma." (Neuroblastoma is a cancer originating in the nervous system that afflicts young children.)

"The use of autologous transplantation in the leukemias is a bit more problematic. The first and therefore longest example of its use is in a disease known as CALLA positive ALL." This is the illness and specific treatment for which Rappeport recommended—with assurance but internal and then projected distress—that the parents take their child to another medical center, the one that was most experienced in the appropriate technique. "The bone marrow was treated with monoclonal antibody directed against CALLA. The information that's available now suggests that the process is of no value in those patients who have relapsed early. And early keeps getting redefined. It has been of value in patients who have relapsed late, but may be of no more value than intensive chemotherapy alone.

"In acute myelogenous leukemia, the bone marrow has been purged with chemotherapeutic agents. The initial reports were extremely enthusiastic. They continued to deteriorate with further reporting. It's my feeling that the information that will come out of those kinds of autologous transplants is that you will have had a shift to the right in the survival curves. That is, you will have given intensive chemotherapy, and the patients will remain disease-free for a longer period of time, but they will ultimately have a relapse." He says it's hard to know for sure. But he says reports from various centers have been highly—even wildly—variable. And of course, he is careful and concerned to say in the spring of 1991, understanding and therapies do change and can improve anytime.

"Autologous transplantation in chronic myelogenous leukemia—that is, where the patients have had their bone marrows frozen when in the stable phase, and then administered to them after intensive treatment of blast crisis—has been of virtually no value because there's been no effective therapy for blast crisis—in either transplantation or nontransplantation."

In Rappeport's description, there is no mention of gene transfer, because although an understanding of its possibility lies in the proven mechanics of transplantation, and the methodology of some of it would be the same as for an autologous transplant, it isn't yet a therapy at his command. He's sure it's only a matter of time until

it will be, but at the moment he's talking about reasonable treatment in the here and now.

"I'd never forgive myself for not having tried," Jane Anderson
Morse said in 1989, a week before Christmas. Her bone marrow
had already been harvested, and she was scheduled to return to the
hospital for her autologous transplant shortly after the first of the
year. Jane is a tall blond with blue eyes, a mellifluous voice, tremendous verve, a remarkably high intelligence, and a spiritual life
that dominates and pervades all her other qualities. She also has an
unusual medical history. She has had both Hodgkin's and non-
Hodgkin's lymphoma, but they are different diseases.

There was a twenty-seven-year hiatus between her bouts, and
although Rappeport says, "It's interesting, from a purely speculative point of view—the Hodgkin's in such a remote past with lymphoma recurring in basically the same area," there is probably no
connection between them. But Brian Smith says, "There's probably something about Hodgkin's or about you [the physiology of a
person afflicted with Hodgkin's] that allows you to get lymphoma.
Hodgkin's leads to a profound T-cell deficiency. And so, like people who have had GVH, or T-cell depletion, or like Wiskott-
Aldrich patients, Hodgkin's patients are immunosuppressed and
therefore more likely to get non-Hodgkin's lymphoma. It's possible
Jane has been immunosuppressed for over twenty-five years."

In 1961 eighteen-year-old Jane Anderson's boyfriend, necking
with her in the parking lot of Marblehead's Eastern Yacht Club—a
blueblood bastion that defines Jane's environment but does not give
a true impression of her character—asked her if one side of her neck
wasn't bigger than the other. Jane said, "No, I don't think so," but
that night she went home and looked in the bathroom mirror, and
sure enough there was some swelling on the right side of her neck
and in the area above her collarbone. She went to a doctor, who
suggested that a surgeon check her, "and so the Sunday that my
parents were bringing me to college—what was then called Connecticut College for Women—for the first time, I stopped at Salem
Hospital [Salem abuts Marblehead] in Massachusetts, and saw Dr.
Thompson, who was a surgeon. He looked at me, and said, 'I think
we should biopsy this in a week, but go ahead and go to orientation,
and come back and we'll biopsy this and see what's happening.'

"I really knew very little about what was going on. I suppose
maybe subconsciously I knew something, but my parents had de-

cided that they really didn't want to frighten me with what was actually happening. My mother did ask him on the way out, 'Could this be malignant?' and apparently he said yes, and obviously my parents were thrown into an incredible tailspin, but they elected to keep as much of the scary news away from me as possible. I came back, had the biopsy, and of course the news was bad, but all I was told was, 'Well, this is something that people your age can get, and we're going to give you some treatments, but everything's going to be fine.' And the treatments amounted to radiation five days a week, Monday through Friday, for four weeks. Also at Salem Hospital."

There was really, as Jane describes it, nothing to it. She drove herself over to the hospital, received X-ray treatments directed at her neck, got up from the table, and drove herself home. She never felt nauseated or sick in any other way, and after a month she returned to school, still ignorant of the danger she had been in and presumably still was.

"When I tell people that, the tendency is for them to be really shocked that my parents wouldn't tell me what was happening. In retrospect, though, I think that probably, knowing myself as I do, that was a wise move at the time. They really thought this would throw me for a loop. And I think if I had known, I might have been completely terrorized. And the fact that I really didn't know what was happening meant that after a month of radiation treatments I went back to college and had a total ball for myself—went to mixers at Wesleyan and Yale, and was the consummate live-it-up college freshman. It was my first time away from home, and I had such a great time. I think if I had found out right away it really could have been harmful.

"In January my boyfriend—the same one who had discovered it—took me out to dinner, and he just sort of let slip that, well, you know, you had cancer. So that's when I really was first aware of it, because my godmother had said something to him, and I guess he wasn't sure that it was still being kept from me. And I went wild! It was still difficult for my mother particularly to talk about it, and she really would hedge a lot. It took a number of years until I finally knew definitively what was going on."

Staging procedures hadn't been established at the time Jane had Hodgkin's disease, but Rappeport says that judging from the treatment she received and its efficacy, she must have had stage I. After the X-ray treatment she was free of disease, but in 1968, when—having married Clay Morse, a navy man, two years earlier—she was pregnant with her first child, her obstetrician "really insisted that we get the records from Salem Hospital. And that's when I first really knew—for sure, in black and white—what had happened."

Jane says her husband Clay was never worried about her medical history. "By the time we got married, I was pretty much past the five-year limit," she says. "The subject would come up from time to time. When I would go for my checkups, Clay wouldn't say a whole lot, but he was thinking, 'Oh God, I hope it's okay,' and he was always concerned that we get a good report. Sometimes I think he is really deeply worried and concerned but isn't showing it. And maybe that's because he's an engineer or he just has a different way of dealing with reality.

"One of the good offshoots of this," having had Hodgkin's disease, and recovered, in the early 1960s, "was that I became a medical curiosity, and doctors always wanted to see me, so I never had problems getting good physicals. Under the military health plan, dependents were not entitled to have physicals at all. You had to go out and get your own, but I never had trouble getting good medical care because they were always very curious about me. 'Oh, you had Hodgkin's. Well! Let's take a look at you.' I did survive with very few medical or physical problems, for twenty-seven years."

"Most of the non-Hodgkin's lymphomas," says Brian Smith, "derive from the B lymphocyte as opposed to the T lymphocyte. The B-cell non-Hodgkin's lymphomas come in two principal flavors. They come in what we used to call favorable lymphoma and what we used to call unfavorable lymphoma. These aren't great terms because 'favorable'— 'Bad,' 'worse,' and 'worst' is really what they should be called. But anyway, people go on for seven, eight, nine years with 'favorable' lymphomas. Often without treatment. Sometimes with treatment. In the very old days, nobody treated them. And then some treatments came along, like chemotherapy, and so all of a sudden everybody started to treat everything that came along. It took a number of years for everyone to realize that although they hated cancer more than they loved life and they really wanted to beat on this tumor, in fact all you did was shorten people's survival or make them miserable or both." How or when to treat this classification of lymphoma still isn't clear, says Smith. "Every time there's a new treatment available, everybody tries to treat people aggressively again." It is, he says, a lot like CML—chronic myelogenous leukemia—in that the disease can lie dormant for years and then explode; the difference between "favorable" lymphomas and CML is that the proliferation of the former is even more unpredictable than that of the latter. "What's odd about them is that although they're favorable, they're the lymphomas that you can't cure; they're 'favorable' because the natural history of them, untreated, is much better than the unfavorable.

"The unfavorable lymphomas are truly unfavorable. In fact, you die within six months of getting the lymphoma, usually, if it goes untreated." But, Smith says, treatment for unfavorable lymphomas followed the development of successful treatment for Hodgkin's disease, and it does work nowadays, about a third to a half of the time. Those therapies, however, did not work for favorable lymphomas.

"There seems to be something paradoxical about it, but what we always say is, It kind of makes sense, because the unfavorable lymphomas are the ones that grow the most rapidly, and are therefore the most sensitive to the kinds of treatments we have these days, which are primitive approaches to trying to kill cells that are dividing like crazy. That's all we know how to do. We don't know a lot, but we know how to kill cells that are growing like crazy. And that's presumably why that group can be treated.

"In any case, it's interesting—there's obviously a basic biological difference between the two. They're derived from the same kinds of cells [B cells] and in many respects they look the same. The fact that the favorable lymphomas will wax and wane, and sometimes when you get a viral infection will go away for a little while, would suggest that they are somehow under immune control. And that's very interesting. The question is, How do you find out what it is that's keeping them under control? What is it that changes either in those cells themselves or in your ability to control them—i.e., your immune system—that allows them to go crazy after five or six or seven years?

"I think it's a better model than trying to look at lung cancer or something else that's uniformly going to kill somebody off in a brief period of time. Because in a way lymphomas are malignant but premalignant conditions at the same time. CML is a very similar issue. You can say all the things I'm saying about the lymphomas about CML. Except the lymphomas are easier to track, just because of the nature of the cell they come from. Eighty-five to 90 percent of them come from B cells. And since B cells don't actually represent the majority of your lymphocytes, it suggests that the change in the cell isn't a sort of random process of your lymphocytes but that it's something about the B cells. And we know that in the normal immune system the T cells control the B cells.

"If you *profoundly* immunosuppress somebody, as you do with a bone marrow transplant, sometimes what will happen is that you will get lymphomas developing. And in particular you will get B-cell lymphomas. They're terrible diseases to treat, for logical reasons. I mean, what is supposed to be keeping them under control is your immune system, but you don't have one, and we don't know how to give you that. We can give you an antibody, but we can't give you T cells."

In fact, says Smith, it's his work with T-cell depletion that got him interested in lymphomas. "I think the bone marrow transplant story, like AIDS, like severe combined immunodeficiency, like Wiskott-Aldrich syndrome—all of which are predispositions to develop lymphomas, all of which are prelymphoma conditions, if you will—I think all of them are trying to tell us something about normal immune control. I think they're telling us that the immune system is in fact effective at keeping tumors under control. The problem is, we don't know what exactly it is. We don't know how to take advantage of it. I think we'll figure it out. I don't know if it will be ten months or ten years or what."

The type of lymphoma with which Jane Morse was afflicted almost three decades after she'd been cured of Hodgkin's disease was what Rappeport describes as one of "the obligatory intermediate types," being neither indolent nor aggressive, not exactly falling into either the "favorable" or "unfavorable" classifications Smith gives. But finding out she had it at all was not easy for Jane, because her concerns were, at first, dismissed. This fact makes her angry, and it makes me furious. It reminds me of Roberta's internist, who dismissed her complaints, thus greatly contributing to the probability she would die. But my anger stems also, as I think Jane's does, from the attitude of many doctors toward women.

From the time she knew about her Hodgkin's, Jane says, "I was concerned about whether there might be some hereditary connection, although no one in my family had ever had Hodgkin's. I think right now that people don't feel that there is a hereditary connection, but it hasn't been ruled out as far as I know. I was always concerned, and still am, about any lump that one of the children might get. During my first year of graduate school [at Yale, where Jane is getting her Ph.D; she was already a priest], in the fall of 1986, my daughter had had a lump in her neck, a small lump, for about nine months. I had taken her to a total of seven doctors, one of whom treated me very rudely. I brought Sarah in and presented her to this physician, and was told in no uncertain terms that I was overreacting and that nodes pop up in kids' necks and that's that."

Another doctor, however, said, "Gee, if this was my daughter I'd have it biopsied." "I was in a rage," Jane says. "I thought, I have taken this child to these people, and they've all said this is nothing, and now you're telling me why didn't I have it biopsied. So I did. And I went through three weeks of absolute terror. She was a senior in high school—seventeen—and it turned out it was benign. Thank God.

"But that's why I have a lot of sympathy for my mother, because even now, I keep saying to myself, At least it's not one of the children that it's happening to. And I do mean that. In some ways it's easier for me to deal with this because it's happening to me. That experience with wondering about Sarah was really one of the bleakest hells I've ever lived through."

In November 1987, a year after this experience with her daughter, Jane's symptoms appeared. She remembers the date exactly—November 11—because she was to celebrate Holy Communion at Berkeley Divinity School and did so despite a fever and swollen nodes in her neck. "Anytime I've noticed swelling in my neck I get hyper." And so when the fever went away but the swelling remained, she went to a local doctor. He put her on antibiotics but said that with her history, Jane should get checked by an ear, nose, and throat specialist.

She did so, and the doctor "seemed virtually unconcerned. But said, 'Well, let's try another antibiotic.' We did that. Nothing happened. I went back, saw another person in that ENT group, here in New London. And after several tries I finally said, 'I think we really ought to biopsy this thing.' But the doctor seemed reluctant to do that. He said, 'I really don't think that this is a problem.' I also went somewhere else, to see another doctor, just to get a second opinion, and was pretty much told, 'Hey, you could have this node for a long time. I've had a node in my neck that size for nineteen years and nothing's changed.'

"Again, I was pretty much patted on the head. This part

makes me extremely angry," Jane says. "The paternalism was so unbelievably unbounded. I just hate that. In both cases my problems were treated very cavalierly." Finally in January of 1988, she did have the lump biopsied at the local hospital and eventually— "there was dillydallying with the report, and that made me mad"— got the diagnosis. "They said it was atypical hyperplasia. Which meant that there was something odd about the structure of the cells. But it was not sufficiently defined to be called malignant. And I was greatly relieved."

Still the nodes remained swollen; Jane thinks they may have gotten larger. In August she went to St. Louis, to Clay's high school reunion, and when she came back, she says, "there was some blockage in my ear, which I first thought was caused by the plane, but when it didn't go away after two weeks, I thought, This is a little odd," and she went to another ENT specialist.

"Dr. Gardiner looked at my neck, and did some other tests with a fiber optic endoscope, and although she was very noncommittal about my previous care—and I think that's typical of doctors, they don't want to bad-mouth other people—my impression was that she was quite shocked, and she said, 'I really think we ought to get you in for a biopsy.' All the while trying to be very calm, and keep me calm. She did say, 'There is a possibility that what is going on here is non-Hodgkin's lymphoma.' Again, it took a long, long time to get the results. I got to the point—after three weeks—when I thought, Gee, it's taken so long and I haven't heard anything; surely everything must be okay."

It was September. Jane returned to Virginia Seminary for convocation, held across the street from the school in the larger Temple Beth El. Between lectures, she went out to a pay phone and called Dr. Gardiner. "And she said, 'You've got lymphoma.' And we talked very briefly about where I could be treated." Dr. Gardiner recommended a doctor at Yale–New Haven Hospital, and said she would set up an appointment.

Jane hung up the phone "and bumped into a couple of my classmates, and one professor who I hardly knew at all, but who had been there when I was in seminary, and we went back into the temple."

Here, Jane cries. As she told me her story, Jane consistently and exclusively cried when telling me that other people cared about her. "I knelt down, and they put their hands on me, and I remember looking up, and instead of what I would usually see on the wall, which would be a cross, I saw this beautiful tree of life. And that stuck in my mind. The first thing I thought was, 'Thank you, God, that I heard this when I heard it, and I've got these friends around to be with me.'

"And they prayed with me. My friends at the seminary used to call me 'the Jewish girl' anyway, because I love Hebrew, and I love that temple, and so there I was. And the beauty of the thing was that within the next few hours, before I got on the plane to come back up, I was able to talk to classmates and professors, and tell them what had happened, and then immediately the prayer network got started. I immediately got on prayer lists, and people were so concerned. I felt from the beginning that I was being upheld by these people, who really loved me."

But she does not at all believe that people bring illness on themselves. "I think that's utter bullshit. I don't know how you can look at a three-month-old baby who has leukemia and say that child is responsible for the disease. But there are lots of people for whom that is the bottom line. That you caused it. There's even stuff in the Bible, in the Biblical tradition, that it's something to do with our sin, that sin brings on ill health. But I think from a Biblical perspective what we're really talking about is a kind of structural sin, that, yes, humankind did screw up the world, when given this wonderful gift by God, but it's because of this huge kind of corporate centralness and the fact that we did screw it up. It's not the way God intended it to be. God didn't want us to have ill health. Theologically it's an extremely difficult problem. You still have to say, Well, if God is powerful enough to do these things, why doesn't God enter in? And I think that's because God has given us the freedom from the very beginning—God isn't a robot manipulator or a puppeteer."

Jane sighs. "I guess what I'm trying to say in sort of flaky theological terms is that I think life is, always has been, and is always going to be a mystery. I think there are a lot of things we simply don't know about God. My thoughts are not your thoughts. I think it's highly presumptuous of us to say that we know how God operates all the time.

"I think that maybe because of my encounter with Hodgkin's, I am an especially incarnational person. I want to be around here. I want to live physically, and I'm not ready for this other-side business yet." Jane talks emotionally about her wishes for the future: to teach, probably at a seminary rather than in a university, because the latter requires detachment, "and I'm just not a detached person." She is eager to impart her love of Hebrew, of the Bible, of spiritual life to other people. She loves her husband and mother, and wants to live for them. Most of all, she wants to live for her children. She wants to see them married—she has always dreamed of performing the ceremonies—and she wants to baptize their babies. She says she was a wild kid, and she claims to be full of faults now, but she is sure she still has a lot to do and to give.

"I think there is something beautiful planned," says Jane. "I just don't know what that is."

In 1988, when Jane was diagnosed, the main thing she remembers finding out was that her particular type of lymphoma was not one of the easiest to treat. Jill Lacy, the oncologist at Yale–New Haven Hospital to whom Dr. Gardiner had sent Jane, "was very clear," Jane says, "and very much concerned that I understood, that my chances were not as good as if it were a more aggressive form." But treatment had, Jane understood, about a 50 percent chance of working, so she started chemotherapy.

It went smoothly. Jane did not get violently sick, and although she was apprehensive about each new test—bone marrow aspirations, CAT scans, MRIs (magnetic resonance imaging, another sophisticated diagnostic tool, similar to a CAT scan and, like it, painless)—and treatment, her fears weren't borne out. She did mind her hair falling out and minded more the puffiness and weight gain the steroids that were part of her protocol provoked, but in February Jane had a CAT scan that showed she was responding remarkably well to the treatments. "They did a couple more CAT scans, and then in April I stopped the chemotherapy," she says. "It looked as if the chemo had done its job, and technically speaking I was declared to be in complete remission. Well, that part of things was all very good, and I was excited to be finished with the chemo. But on one of those CAT scans, they had picked up something at the base of my skull which they thought might possibly be an aneurysm. I did not handle that very well at all. I thought, Good God, I've been through this, I've finally— And I'm told, 'By the way, you might have an aneurysm.' So I really—I was beginning to wonder how much more— And if one more person came up to me and said"—Jane speeds up her normal voice and adds a nasal twang—" 'The Lord never gives you any more than you can handle,' " she says, echoing Peter Lariviere, "I was going to spit, shit and any other bodily thing I could do that was offensive. But Dr.

seriously—if I worked myself into such a state of fear that in some sense I let myself open for it to come back. I really don't believe this. But I got to the point where—as much as I think this is actually hogwash—I would be worried about how I was praying, what I was asking for. I'd think, Jesus, Jane! Do you really believe in a God who is going to give cancer to you if you don't say the words in the right order? I mean, I've never believed that! But these thoughts would come to me."

For an autologous transplant, Rappeport says, "the risks are different" from what they are for an allogeneic transplant. "Recurrences of the underlying disease, if it's for a malignancy, are greater in the autologous rather than in an allogeneic. Obviously the risk of GVH is less." But "the medication risks are exactly the same. The preparative regimen is exactly the same. The immunosuppressive risks are for a shorter period of time, and they seem to be less severe."

And so Jane's hospitalization was much like the others I've described, except that she is herself—just as Wesley, and Peter, and Ricky, and Daniel, and Jennie, and everyone else are all different from one another, also. The only real procedural difference is that since Jane was her own donor, the marrow—after an aspiration indicated no detectable malignancy—was taken from her rather than from another person and frozen and, several weeks later, after she had undergone standard chemotherapeutic preparation for a transplant, reinfused. She was not irradiated, because her old medical records were unobtainable and so Rappeport didn't know how much radiation she had received when she was treated for Hodgkin's and therefore how much she could tolerate now.

Jane had two brief hospitalizations before the transplant, so that her response to the chemotherapeutic drugs to be used more intensively in the transplant process itself could be tested; these were trying and troubling for her, because both times her hospital room—not on the bone marrow transplant unit—was filthy. The first time, a refrigerator in her room had been defrosted, and the floor was wet and slippery. During the second, which lasted four days, the toilet was never cleaned, and both she and her roommate suffered from diarrhea. It was not only a disgusting problem but a worrying one, because both women had suppressed immune systems. Jane, tactful and generous in every instance, allows that it is difficult to get people to clean, but also says I can quote her on these

Lacy was very good about getting me in to get an MR
and it turned out it was nothing.

"I did go back to the clinic for a checkup again, an
also saw Dr. Gardiner again, my ear, nose, and throat d
she did a fiber optic endoscope exam of my nasopharyn
areas that were affected originally in the diagnosis we
sopharynx and nodes in my left neck. And she said that
was absolutely clear. So that's the point at which I beg
back into my work. I'd go up to the Connecticut Colleg
with my L. L. Bean bookbag stuffed to the gills, and
excited about memorizing my paradigms. And I really w
ing full steam ahead with trying to get ready for compre
But as the summer wore on, things turned out not to be

By August, a CAT scan showed the disease had recu
that began the new Reign of Terror. And I have since
talked to so many doctors that it's almost a blur, with
happened."

Jane went to the Memorial Sloan-Kettering Cancer C
New York to get another opinion. She talked to Dr. Lacy,
weighed her alternatives. "By the end of September my
and I together had reached a decision that we were com
with. That, even though the transplant was the scariest t
was the only thing in which the word 'cure' was realistic to
with. And I don't want to just buy time.

"My daughter," says Jane, "was really scared. About to
and things. And I think if she had her way, she would lik
me deal with this completely through diet—namely, macrol
Because she's so afraid of what may happen to me in the pro
trying to wipe out the cancer. So it's been very hard for he

Clay Morse believes in healing through prayer; in the
on of hands.

"Clay and I made the decision together," Jane says
transplant. "I certainly consider myself open to all kinds of tl
I've been interested in how macrobiotic diets can help, either
prevention—or some people claim to be cured by that. But
have enough faith in Western medicine, and also am enough
Westerner, to think there are some serious problems with son
the claims made or some of the demagoguery that goes on.

"One of the issues that came up for me spiritually, after I
told I was in remission, is that I lived in so much fear every day
the disease would come back. I almost wonder—not tot

complaints. When I do so to Rappeport, he is thin-lipped with anger—at the filth, not at Jane. She was relieved at the cleanliness of the transplant unit.

Jane found visitors helpful, especially "ones who don't presume to understand. People who care enough to get mad that this is happening to you help the most." The isolation, she says, "is not as nice a one as I had thought." Jane had expected that as a scholar accustomed to working alone, she wouldn't mind the laminar flow room too much, but she often felt, she says, "like a specimen."

The physical environment was ugly, too, and there was a lot of noise—clanking and banging, even at night. "I love animals and plants—not having them was a real deprivation. And not being able to touch people or hug them. So much of what I perceive as being human was denied me. For good reason, but it was hard." Sometimes she would take naps. "Not because I was tired, but to shut out the noise and turmoil going on around me." It was hard to get comfortable enough to read, because she suffered from rectal infection and irritation. Listening to music helped the most. She would have liked to watch TV, but the quality of sound was grating. Most of all, "I wanted to go home so badly I could taste it."

Once home, Jane said she was grateful everything had gone so well, but she was "living from CAT scan to CAT scan. It doesn't get any easier." She does not want to hear—and never did want to hear—doomsayers. "It ruins your whole day when you're trying to make a comeback."

"I was determined," says Clay, "to support Jane in whatever she wanted. And it was clear that of the medical ways, bone marrow transplant was the best. It's very hard. You're the husband, you want to support the person. If it was me, I'd go the whole-health route [nontraditional medicine], but it's not me. Once you understand bone marrow transplant—and most people don't understand the whole concept—it's the best of the medical options." Clay is tall, broad-shouldered, heavyset.

Clay loves Jane. He talks about getting up at four in the morning to juggle bills. He talks about developing a better relationship with his wife taking her for clinic visits. He talks about being very hurt when, after months of closeness, a five-minute argument created a weeks-long rift. He talks about the differences between himself and his wife. Clay insists his actions bespeak his feelings. Jane, he says, tries to interpret his emotions by reading his facial expression. He finds this grossly unfair. Though his point is specific and his trouble piercing, his description sounds so familiar I almost laugh: it is the same argument my husband and I have been having for almost twenty years.

"My advice to anyone," says Clay Morse, "is if the doctors say three weeks, wait three weeks. Don't read into it, don't look at body language or anything. Jane was depressed when she had her last CAT scan, because she thought the expression on one of the nurses' faces meant something. But it came back fine. In our family we all know each other. We can look at personality traits qualitatively and with a sense of humor. I know I talk with a lot of detachment," Clay says—a statement I found strikingly untrue. "I don't want to get knocked for that."

The preparation for each hospital visit was so anxiety-provoking that it would become, for Clay, a relief to get Jane into the hospital each time. "I try to go through this with Jane, and feel with her. But it would become such a relief. Like in the navy"—Clay Morse now has his own consulting business, but for a long time he was the commanding officer of a submarine—"there's relief when the ship is under way. You prepare, and then you leave. To me it was like you pull in the anchor—pull in the line—and she's in the hospital."

When she was about to get out of the hospital, Clay says, there was the question of the cats. Jane loves their cats, but cats carry germs. "One thing I like about Dr. Rappeport is he's very conservative on the cleanliness thing. I sound like George Bush, 'the cleanliness thing.' Anyway, I wanted to get rid of the cats—not kill them, put them on farms. Then, at a meeting, Dr. Rappeport said, 'If the cats are important to Jane, we have to work it out.' And I appreciate that." In fact, though the Morses wouldn't have known it, Rappeport hates cats. "And the cats *are* important to Jane," Clay says. "So we worked something out." The "something" they "worked out," Clay reports, resulted in "cat damage to the attic. But Jane did get to see her cats."

There has been dissension and disturbance within the family. Sarah and Ben are both unusually bright and sensitive young people, devoted to their mother. Jane's illness and the treatment for it are depressing and troubling for them, but they too have faith. Bad feeling grew, for the first time, between Clay and Jane's mother. "That's the fallout from this thing," Clay says. "But it's her daughter who's sick, and I have to understand that.

"I do think this last year Jane and I have gotten a lot closer. We were always close, but we're a lot more aware now of our own weaknesses."

"We won't know for years," says Jane, "whether it's a cure."

"Jane and I," says Clay, "want to enjoy and live life." It is the summer, six months after Jane's transplant.[5] Clay and Sarah have both been in a local production of *Fiddler on the Roof*. "Jane went to all four performances," Clay says. "And at the cast party we danced every dance and sang every song. We grasp the moment more. That's the beauty of it."

Even in the hospital, Jane says, "I never felt totally cut off from God, but I did reach a point when I found it hard to pray. I ended up relying on other people to pray for me. I'd say God's name, and then they'd take over. That was something I had to learn. I've always been very independent—one of those who thought I had to do everything or it would fall apart. That's not a good way to be, if you're a priest. You are a part of the community—the broad circle of God's people. I don't think I knew what it was to be part of God's body. I see more of the blessing of being part of a community of faith than I did before; I don't see how I could have gotten through it without it. We churchgoers are just as lousy as everyone else, but we band together to do God's will." Jane thinks suffering and prayer are related, and, she says happily, she'll get to more of that when she writes her dissertation. "It was hard to feel sorry for myself when so many people around me were showing love and concern, and thus showing God's love."

"When you ask me about Patrick's faith," Nancy Thompson said to me, "or about what he said that made him the person he was—I don't know, it's just the way he was. It was the way he related to people. A lot of people will comment to me, staff people will say, 'I'll never forget the way he laughed. His smile. The way his shoulders jiggled when he got a kick out of something.' And those are the things that people remember."

One time before her transplant, Jane Morse says, Brian Smith came into a clinic examination room. "Dr. Rappeport said, 'This is Dr. Smith. He's always threatening me about going back to Princeton and doing a degree in philosophy, which is sort of like what you're interested in.' I made some kind of remark, and we laughed. And that was the extent of my encounter with him [Smith] then. But my impression of him was someone I could really talk to. Just the way he laughed when I was fresh, you know, I thought he was a good person." And of Rappeport Jane says, every time I talk to her, "He's a prince."

There must be atheists who have bone marrow transplants, but as it happens I haven't met them. Everyone who talked to me about his or her experience believed in God, and only a few blamed Him. I do not doubt that it is human error and the current inadequacy of knowledge that failed the people I've written about who died, and that science and medicine and nursing care saved those who survived. And yet the trials and effort it's been my privilege to listen to and witness and try to describe seem to me to transcend—in their very embodiment of the value of the individual—any single life. The paradox is the stuff of psalms.

"You find God," says the Reverend Jane Morse, "through the incarnational people around you."

Conclusion

Bill Mason, whose daughter Jill died in 1982, is the man who said Rappeport looks like a beagle. Bill and Jennifer Mason talked to me at the very beginning of my research, agreeing to do so largely because of the great and lasting affection they feel for Rappeport.

"He doesn't mind taking that extra risk with people," Bill says. "It's all well and good to have that idealism when you're ten or twelve years old, but when you're a grown man to still have that instinct, and to be willing to sacrifice yourself, that's an amazing thing to watch.

"What I remember is that he would always center on Jill. And every so often he'd look over his shoulder at pictures of patients and tell a story about one of them in an incredibly encouraging way. He must have spent hours—four straight hours—talking. I've never seen anyone so absolutely driven and committed to his goal."

Jill had aplastic anemia. She was not sick for long and never seemed very sick. In Bill's office, snapshots of Jill are grouped together in a frame. Even those that show her toward the end of her life are of a healthy, wholesome teenager, a tanned, smooth-skinned, and serene almost-woman. Good humor was her hallmark. She was happiness. "We never dreamed," Bill says, "that terminal illness was involved with a child that vibrant."

She died four days into the chemotherapeutic preparation for a bone marrow transplant. As a result of research based partly on her experience, cyclophosphamide, the drug against which her heart reacted, is now administered according to body surface, rather than weight. Jill's weight at death was somehow not recorded on her chart. Two years later, over the phone, Jen supplied it to researchers. "I knew what she weighed when she was born, and what she weighed when she died," Jen says. Momentarily, she lifts her hands from her lap. "A mother."

"You never get over it," she said to me, on another occasion, two years later, after Roberta had died and I was talking about my own mother. "Never." Jen's words could have been those of any of the mothers I've met who have lost children and thus endured the unbearable. But she, like them, still remembers Rappeport as life-giving.

Rappeport blames himself for Jill Mason's death. But "Jill had looked straightforward," he says. He went on vacation, calling in every day. Still, he says, "You always wonder if you'd been there, maybe you'd have thought of something." He came down from New Hampshire to see for himself when Jill had one more day of treatment left before the transplant. If they had stopped the drug, Rappeport explains, she would probably have rejected the graft, and with her immune system gone and her own marrow not functioning she "would have been left with nothing."

According to Jen, "she was able to drink only teaspoons of water." The doctors lowered the dosage of cyclophosphamide, but her kidneys failed, her heart failed. "Everything went," Jen says. "They called us. 'Get in here quick.' The Masons ran through the narrow streets and alleys between their hotel and the hospital. With her hand, Jen shows them swerving. "But she was already gone."

It was two o'clock in the morning of Monday, August 23. Rappeport was there, Jen says. "He came in with all the doctors, and he embraced us." "He was as devastated as we were," says Bill. "It was just that medical science hadn't stretched itself to the frontiers enough to help our daughter. To save our daughter. You could see in his eyes that he was lost.

"It's an extraordinary force. You can play a lot of things safe in life. He doesn't."

*   *   *

Today, Rappeport has constantly increasing resources. The changes, even when the outcome is dramatic, are incremental: there hasn't been a moment in Rappeport's career, nor is there likely to be one, when a single breakthrough, or even a series of clearly linked advances, changes everything. But if we take even a slightly longer view, a lot has happened. Rappeport's patients live now because of drugs and techniques developed during his career—from drugs such as acyclovir to mechanical devices such as Hickman lines to the supersensitive laboratory methods molecular biology has brought. With gene mapping, more is known about the HLA complex, and with molecular biology's technology, testing for HLA compatibility is greatly improved over that available in Ricky Stott's day, or Peter Lariviere's. Hospital stays for bone marrow transplant patients get shorter all the time, and survival rates, when compared with those a couple of decades ago, are miraculous. Progress continues and is accelerating: the growing understanding of disease, particularly at the genetic level, holds out great hope of conquering it.

The specifics add up. Many researchers, including Smith and Rappeport, are working on aspects of cell adhesion, trying to figure out more about how cells recognize one another, stick to one another, and communicate with one another. If you could figure out more of this, Smith says, you could get cells to "talk to each other" when they're not but should be. You could also, with different needs, do the opposite: "If you wanted to interfere with graft-versus-host disease," says Smith, "or graft rejection, maybe what you should do is interfere with the ability of the host and donor cells to find each other. Or with their ability to know that they've found each other. That's what the thrust of cell-adhesion work is." It's less than five years old, and still speculative.

The growth factors, though, have moved from the laboratory to the clinic, promising fast cellular recovery in people who will die if their bodies do not quickly start manufacturing blood components. Some of these substances are now proven and licensed, others are still being tested, and still more are in the developmental stage. Fetal cord blood, already a lifesaving source in some instances, may become more widely used. For some genetic diseases apparent in fetuses, in utero transplants of stem cells may become common practice.

The pool of unrelated donors may expand, and its use may become more effective and efficient. Donor registries, unavailable to Patrick Thompson, are now going concerns, but it is still difficult to come up with a match, although there are long lists of volunteers and widespread publicity about the need for them. Unrelated donors have been used for only a short time, and so the long-term effects aren't known, but such a match certainly seems like salvation for anyone who needs a donor but has no suitable relative. And because bone marrow, unlike hearts and lungs and pancreases and kidneys, regenerates, the supply of donors is, at least theoretically, unlimited. Furthermore, whatever problems do reveal themselves in transplants between unrelated donors are likely to be amenable to the correction that research into the problems of more conventional matching provides.

Today, a half match from a relative, a better match from someone outside the family, and the use of one's own presumably disease-free marrow ("hopefully, disease-free," says Brian Smith) are in the vanguard of an up-to-the-minute hematologist's armory. They are not, however, uniformly usable. Beyond them lie possibility: that graft-versus-host disease can be reliably controlled, that the purging of malignant cells from the marrow will become more effective. Smith talks too about "inverse purging"—selecting and isolating the cells needed and transplanting only those, rather than eliminating the undesirable cells; this would be the opposite of leukemia purging, or T-cell depletion. There's a widespread effort to make bone marrow transplants more effective in treatment for people with solid tumors. And always, the critical struggle continues: to understand the mechanics of cell growth and division and interaction well enough to find ways to foil malignancies.

Above all rises hope for therapeutic gene transfer. This developing technology, though part of the scientific/medical continuum, has potential for reaching farther, and radiating more widely, than anything that has been well tested has yet done. Much of the understanding of its possibility comes from bone marrow transplantation. For example, the scientific result of Daniel Folsom's transplant is the knowledge that introduction of healthy tissue through one set of cells—hematopoietic stem cells—can and will positively affect other damaged and malfunctioning ones. With gene transfer, patients without a donor could be cured through extracting, changing, and reinserting their own bone marrow or cells of their skin or other organs, or through manipulation of blood cells. Techniques similar to those proposed for hereditary disease may be used against cancer, heart disease, and AIDS, but this hasn't really happened yet. Gene therapy hasn't yet been *proved* efficacious in human beings, and its very glamour could diminish the realization of its full possibility.

At the end of the twentieth century, the greatest promise for the cure of terrible illness lies in understanding and manipulating genes. Huge sums of money back the research, and glory awaits those who are the first to achieve—or seem to achieve—dramatic results. In 1991, experiments at the National Institutes of Health on people dying of cancer and on children born with a particular kind of SCID—adenosine deaminase (ADA) deficiency—have a high visibility. They seem miraculous. And they are, in the sense that the abstract made concrete always is. Paradoxically, however, it is the cautionary voices that seem the most passionate and persuasive.

The loudest of these—in my ear—is Richard Mulligan's, the basic scientist whose expertise is in gene transfer. He is highly critical of the experiments at NIH, and that, combined with both the fact is that by speaking out he opens himself to accusations of greed and envy, and that he seems to believe gene therapy will ultimately be able to cure anything and everything, are a lot of what convinces me. Mulligan is a true believer who wants to hold back, wants to wait until the value of what he—and other scientists— have found and are finding can be seen clearly. His combination of passion and restraint helps persuade me of his integrity. There is also the length and single-mindedness of his effort: His work is transduction—getting a missing or altered gene into a cell that will carry it to its working location—and he's been at it for over a decade, with no sign of letup. His dedication to one aspect of a critically important field with tremendous potential application echoes that of Max Perutz.

In this, he's also like his colleague Frank Grosveld, who has labored over the globin gene and continues to do so in the same way, with the result that he's able to say, "This lab knows just about everything about globin delivery." He's also the developer of a sickle cell mouse, a great achievement that allows research to advance in this widespread and devastating disease. One pictures such scientists crouched over petri dishes and microscopes and—these days—in front of computer screens, but that isn't where or how I saw them. Grosveld in particular was open-eyed and sociable, regularly going off into tangents on subjects of easy human accessibility. He talked about in vitro fertilization, using it as an example of high-tech medicine that is "not a piece of cake" but in fact "a very traumatic experience" for the woman; he's cautioning against an understanding of experimental therapy as an easy solution.

On the subject of sickle cell anemia, there is the gratification in talking to groups of lay people afflicted with the disease, of seeing how much they want to understand, and can. "You can explain almost anything to these people, because they're so interested." Nevertheless, again, despite his hope in gaining information leading to the cure, he himself—as things stand right now—is in favor of prenatal testing and abortion for the terrible diseases with which he's concerned. "Prevention is the best way to go." But "parental choice, medical advice, who decides is very important." And then, clarifying my understanding of his comments, "Parental choice is the *most* important" factor in decision making. "In communities where such programs are in operation, even conservative, very religious [Catholic] people clearly choose pro screening and pro termination of pregnancy. This has been documented for Sardinia and Cyprus."[1]

Richard Mulligan also is aware of the suffering catastrophic illness brings. That is why he argues for restraint, saying that if there's premature application of theory to human beings, false results will ensue. "I think one thing you ought to look into," he said to me, "is whether there really is a difference between the scientist and the clinician in terms of wanting to go faster or do things quicker. The reason I say that is I think it's very misunderstood by people. I mean, I feel like I couldn't be more practical. I couldn't want things to go faster. I'm not in my ivory tower just scratching my head. But as a scientist I feel there's a certain rigor in anything I would do."

It's important to listen to what he's saying, because he's stating a scientist's humanitarianism. He's saying *more* people will suffer if a capitulation to desperation involves cutting corners. "I always look at it as if my wife or mother had cancer, would I want them to get this—you know—some newfangled approach. That's the best way to look at it, I think. If there is some reasonable chance of benefit, I think it's worthwhile trying. The problem is that the science can disappear so quickly when you use the emotion of 'Well, people are dying! We have to do something!' The worry is not so much that you're going to hurt people by doing this. *It's just that you're going to miss what's important.* You're going to take a track that's not going to get you there. Or it may get you there in fact much slower, even though the process is in force."

The italics are mine. I have emphasized Mulligan's words because I think with them he answers people who doubt that the expense and anguish of human experimentation are worth it. Yes, he says, if someone is dying and anything might help, it's reasonable to use it. But be clear on what you can learn from doing so. Experiment is not a dirty word, even when the subject is human. The critical point is not to shy away from human experimentation, thinking it's awful and pretending it's something else, but instead to define each experiment's terms properly, just as one would in a procedure carried out in a test tube or on a mouse. Doing so doesn't take away from a patient being honestly dealt with and kindly treated; on the contrary, truthfulness is a necessary component of decency. I think Mulligan's voice is important because he states a reality that has to be included in a definition of compassion in cutting-edge medicine if it is to meld with science as it should.

Mulligan is straightforward in saying that the specific clinician/basic scientist comparison he's drawing is between himself and the doctors at the NIH who are, in his opinion and that of others, moving ahead too quickly and without proper controls, because they are allowing bright media lights to diminish the clarity of their direction and view.

I don't think the correct contrast is between people of different occupations, between basic scientists versus doctors. Instead, I think he's right in the implicit generalization with which he continues, as he goes on to say the validity of the effort and the truth of the results are dependent on the rigor to which he's referred, on the judgment of the individual: "I've often thought, if I got an M.D. in the next five or ten years, it would be very interesting—because I don't believe my viewpoint would change in terms of how to treat a patient and at what point."

It is for astuteness and integrity on this issue that Brian Smith particularly and repeatedly credits Rappeport. Rappeport knows which research possibility, out of dozens, is the one to focus on and stick with, the one from which the most can be learned and the largest number of people saved. "I think Joel can do a better job of assessing all that than a pure basic scientist," Smith says. "I just think—but I have a prejudice, and it may be because I'm an M.D. and not a Ph.D.—that it gets done *better* from the M.D. side, and

I think that's because in medical school you do learn some basic science, whereas in basic science you don't learn a heck of a lot of medicine."

I can't see any difference between Mulligan's attitude and Rappeport's on research and its applicability; I think it is a matter of character and personality and intelligence, and therefore isn't a question of whether one is a "medic," as Grosveld puts it, or a basic scientist. To help people with whom you're actually faced, as Rappeport does, is surely a virtuous thing. To be interested in what might help them more seems to me necessary not only from an ethical point of view but from an emotional one; despite Rappeport's many successes, most of his patients still die of the diseases that bring them to him.[2] If he were not an exceptionally cautious person to start with, his life's work would certainly have taught him to be: many of the winning and pleading faces he meets are obliterated almost as soon as they're firmly imprinted on his consciousness. Sometimes his treatment kills them—he's fully cognizant of this fact, and it makes him very wary. He doesn't brush aside the possibility of terrible complications years hence, either; the people bearing them will reappear in his office, die in his hospital. How can he, caring as he does, survive if he does not try to think of what else there might be to do?

"I think there's a complex perceptual issue here," Brian Smith says. "The doctors want to do something for somebody who's dying. And I think if they have somebody who's dying and a disease that's going to kill the person no matter what in the next three months, they do tend to say, 'Well, what the hell, let's try this. Because as long as somebody understands what we're doing, you're not going to lose a heck of a lot by trying whatever this is.' But wanting to cure the patient is only one of the motivations for jumping in and doing something when somebody's going to die within the next three months. And I think there are at least two. Motivation one is because you don't want them to die in three months. I think Joel has that motivation. Motivation two is 'Well, if I jump in and do something and it even looks vaguely interesting, I can publish it, and then I'll become a famous doctor.' I don't think that the best clinical researchers are like that at all. I think if you talk to somebody who's good, they're going to say, 'Well, we have an alternative treatment, so we now have to assess this in light of the alternative treatment.'

"When I was first a postdoc in the lab, I remember my boss

saying, 'There's only one person who I've ever been able to get samples from on a patient that ever made any sense, and that's Joel.' And that's because he wouldn't forget it, he would do it, he would be enthusiastic about finding out what the results were, he would modify things if they seemed to need to be modified. I mean, he didn't just want to get a paper out of this. Everybody else wanted to generate one or two samples, and got discouraged if they weren't going to get a paper out of it, or if they realized they were only going to be middle author in a long list of people. But Joel really wanted to know."

"People like that don't change," said Bob Burdett, Rappeport's high school science teacher.

"What gives Joel an international reputation," says Smith, "what has made him a superb clinical investigator, is transplanting two patients, three patients, one patient," as in Gaucher's disease, or Wiskott-Aldrich syndrome, "and combining clinical results with basic science information so you learn what to do for forty patients, thirty patients.

"Joel wants to be famous like everyone else," says Smith, "but I think he spends 90 percent of his time thinking, Well, is this likely to be of benefit to the patient? He'll do something totally outrageous if he thinks the answer to that is yes."

Roberta died September 17, 1989. That summer, my relationship with Rappeport was both strained and sustaining. My sister's leukemia had recurred the previous January, two years after the transplant, and from that time, for her and for those of us close to her, dread was the pivot of existence.

Before that, the transplant had had terrible consequences. Roberta had suffered not only graft-versus-host disease and pneumonia, but also a complication so rare that it was not even included in the encompassing threats of the consent form: she had become paralyzed as a result of excessive radiation. When she was first diagnosed with Hodgkin's disease, which preceded the myelodysplasia that transformed into the leukemia for which she received her transplant, her illness was far advanced—much further, in my family's view, then and now, than it should have been. Roberta had repeatedly, over many months, told her primary-care physician of a bad cough and of fevers that did not abate. He was impatient with her complaints. He did not diagnose cancer, and he did not refer her to appropriate specialists. Finally, months after the onset of symptoms, a surgeon removed tumors from Roberta's groin—gasping, Roberta told me, as he saw them. Still, as with Jane Morse, no doctor took command. Roberta called *him*; she had to initiate the conversation that gave her the information that she had a far-advanced malignancy.

Only then, when a fine hematologist-oncologist took over her care, did she begin to receive proper treatment. It was intensive MOPP therapy and, for the large tumor she then had in her neck—so large it immobilized her arm—a big dose of radiation. She was well for about a year and a half after this time, but both of these necessary therapies caused problems. First, her leukemia is presumed to have resulted from the MOPP regimen. The type of leukemia she had—megakaryocytic leukemia as a second malignancy—could be treated *only* with a bone marrow transplant. At forty-eight, with her disease not in remission, she was a terrible risk, but Rappeport, to whom she was referred at this point, thought she had no chance of living more than a few weeks without a transplant. He worried that because of the dose she'd already received, she would not be able to tolerate total body irradiation, but with the radiologists' counsel and calculations, he decided it was safe to go ahead. This turned out not to be so; the cumulative radiation to her neck invisibly severed her spinal cord. Less than a year after the transplant symptoms appeared: she could not walk, she became incontinent. She was diagnosed as having a radiation-induced myelitis of the upper spine. The paralysis would progress upward, perhaps following a "staggered" course—that is, she would sometimes recover some physical capacity, only to lose that and more—but this new problem would, if she lived the necessary months until it completed its devastation, leave her a quadriplegic, dependent on a respirator.

Everyone was horrified. The radiologists went over and over their calculations, trying to figure out where they'd gone wrong. I was sitting in Rappeport's office at Yale when he, talking on the phone to Roberta's doctor in Boston, found out the problem and told me. I asked him if Roberta would die, and he told me she would, within "a couple of months." I felt my face go cold, a sensation I have never—before or since—experienced. Rappeport asked me if I was all right, if I felt able to drive.

At home, everyone—including and particularly Roberta—was distraught. But we got used to the disability. Roberta didn't die within a couple of months. (No one had given her this prognosis; as

far as I know, only Rappeport saw the situation in those particular terms of bleakness.) Her devoted husband became an expert on aids for the handicapped, home health-care workers managed while he was at work, and Roberta's beloved doctor—Gary Gilliland, a fellow to whom Rappeport had assigned her care when he went to New Haven—tirelessly generated and accompanied the optimism she needed. "I'll take it," was Roberta's conclusion about her radically diminished physical capability.

I want to emphasize that no one in my family, and certainly not Roberta herself, ever blamed Rappeport or any of the doctors who worked with him—including the radiologists who did the calculations—for what happened, nor do we now. All of us were, and remain, grateful to Rappeport for agreeing to perform Roberta's transplant. He did so because of his principles: he will always give a chance at life to someone who wants it. It is not the high-tech physicians who hurt Roberta. If there is anyone to blame—and my mother and brother-in-law and Roberta's four children and I all think there is—it was her original "family" doctor, who by ignoring her symptoms and dismissing her complaints, denied her early, probably curative treatment. I don't know what this man's motives were. I suspect he simply didn't want to be bothered. But the fact is he turned his back on trouble, and by doing so made it worse and probably mandated a tragic outcome. That is the way Roberta saw it, and that is the way I do. And I, as she, remain in Rappeport's debt for the extension of life he gave her. She saw the transplant as a success. It gave her more life than she would otherwise have had, in large ways and small: she saw her daughter married, she read books, listened to the music she loved, saw her friends, talked and talked and talked. I don't agree with Rappeport's statement that partial successes are failures.

Roberta showed herself to be a noble person, of great bravery and endurance and balance, because she had the time—those last couple of years—in which to do so. Extreme medical efforts, done for those who want them, are not harsh and cruel. It is the opposite—it is highly compassionate—to employ even imperfect life-giving means. The willingness to do so and the effort involved are both the embodiment of old-fashioned virtues and the reality of progress.

Roberta did not die from the myelitis. By the spring of 1989 she was visibly bleeding—into her mouth and ears, into her urine, and under her skin, so that huge black bruises showed on her neck

and arms, with smaller petechiae evident, too. A Hickman line had been reimplanted, and she was dependent on transfusions. We waited for the hemorrhage or the infection that was sure to soon take her life, but the apprehension was nothing like normal expectation.

Looking back, I see that there is no reality without hope. I often asked when the end would come, but despite everything, it was unbelievable that Roberta would be gone, because she was here and she wanted to stay. When I went to see her, she talked—over and over again, often using the same phrases, identically, in succession—about the possibility of a cure, about the value of any extension of life, about the fact that, after all, she was "still puttering along." She talked about the possibility of an afterlife, frequently addressing her comments on this subject to my husband, a Catholic. She talked intimately with my mother; I don't know what they said to each other. She talked to her rabbi—a wonderful man who visited often—and when my mother asked what had been said, Roberta replied, "Heavy stuff, Mum."

I talked to Rappeport. Through this time, I was doing my work—that is, I was doing research for this book—and that involved my spending many days in New Haven, following Rappeport around, asking him questions, and seeing his patients. As usual, he was often distracted and impatient, and his irritability was hard to take when I was living through, as well as looking at and listening to, so much trouble and sadness. I am sure he felt guilt over Roberta's myelitis, but the guilt was certainly compounded by relief that she would die, through no fault of his, before her paralysis was complete. I think he turned his feelings back on me, misinterpreting my grief as anger against him.

And he suffered from a mixture of other emotions. I had just signed a publishing contract, making this book a certainty. Though Rappeport very much wanted me to write it, he is unaccustomed to allowing anyone—especially a woman and a nondoctor—control. He sometimes stood in the way of my gathering information I needed: preventing me from going to a scientific meeting Brian Smith had arranged for me to attend, for example, or procrastinating an interview he'd agreed to, and then giving me short, inadequate answers. His self-protectiveness made him cramped and afraid under my scrutiny. Rappeport, though prestigious in his own field, is not a person in public life: he has had no experience as

the subject of a portrait, and didn't, couldn't, gauge how he would feel about it or what the outcome would be. This was worse for him than it would be for most other people, because he is so completely a doctor. My professional role created a seriously disturbing disequilibrium: Rappeport is used to being the one who does the examining. And so I was an outsider, someone with whom he was uneasy and of whom he was mistrustful.

All the same, when in my distress over Roberta's condition I turned to him, he gave help beyond what anyone else could do. He must have heard everything I had to say many times, but just as he had in our first meeting nearly three years earlier, he acted toward me with the particularity Bill Mason describes in Rappeport's behavior toward Jill. I called Rappeport often in July and August and September. He always had time, he always engaged himself in what I had to say. He often said he couldn't answer my questions, that he hadn't examined Roberta recently, that he couldn't predict exactly how the disease would run its course, he couldn't interpret with precision a symptom I reported to him. One time, while talking to him about something else, I added, "and I feel bad about Roberta," and at those words a stream of tears I had no idea was coming fell from my eyes to the table between us (like my face going cold, this was a one-time event), and Rappeport said, "I know." We didn't discuss my emotions. But every time I offered information about Roberta's condition or asked him a question, he explored and explained each point with me, and the energy with which he addressed these physical details told me that Roberta mattered, and that I did.

And again, as he had when I'd first met him, he took away fear. That is, his knowledge, his willingness to share it, and the calm and sad straightforwardness with which he acknowledged the great void in our knowledge that still exists were an additional grace, giving me a companion that made terror recede. Beyond that, the understanding I'd gained from being part of his world gave me confidence in the future: eventually, for the fulfillment of Rappeport's wish that the diseases he treats be eradicated and, in the meantime, for each individual stricken.

Many of the people I met who were dying when they came to Rappeport are alive and well now. And that is because vitality and hope accompany sadness and exhaustion in the medicine Rappeport practices, just as they do in his personality.

*   *   *

My purpose in writing *Life's Blood* has been to show practice in order to influence theory, so that both personal understanding and public policy can better take into account actual experience. Bone marrow transplantation is a prototype of the newest medicine. Here, a technology is shuffling, like Rappeport, just ahead of certain death. With nothing else sure, terror ought to be the only constant. But as Wesley Fairfield said right after his hospitalization, "The hope subdues the fear."

Wesley is now married and, as of the fall of 1991, four years after his transplant, is a Harvard Medical School student. He will be studying a block away from the Patrick Thompson House, the "adult recovery house" to which Nancy referred in her thank-you letter to Rappeport. It is a comfortable place where long-term patients can recuperate near the hospital, and in which their families can stay. The Richard D. Frisbee III Foundation, formed to gather and distribute money in order to care for children afflicted with the diseases bone marrow transplantation addresses, and ultimately to find a cure for them, is also a going concern.

Jane Morse is back at her studies full-time. One day in October, she sits at a seminar table at Yale Divinity School. The room has a parquet floor, cracked in places, a chair rail running along green-painted—and dirt-smudged—walls and, for no discernible reason, a framed, free-standing mirror. Piano music, being played downstairs, is audible, and the view through the window is of a clear, perfect day. The subject under discussion is part of an ongoing scholarly one about the physical environment of a specific group of people, in a particular area, during the time the Jewish Bible—the Old Testament—was being lived. There's nothing arcane about the conversation. It is, after all, perfectly real that people then cooked and housed their animals and traded and traveled and developed. As with all study, you have to know the why in order to figure out the how. Addressing such issues is Jane's business. She's planning to write her thesis on Job, from an existential point of view. "I don't have the answers," she says, "but I want to explore it."

With Rappeport, it's a little different. For him, history is present with more urgency than it is for a scholar. The images of the people I have written about, and many others, press onto and in him, obligating him with their need, and thus giving him his virtue. At Roberta's funeral, my mother put her hand on his shoulder. "Thank you," she said, "for everything you did."

Rappeport shook his head. "We didn't do enough," he said, his voice unsentimental, almost sharp.

"No," said my mother. Her face was covered with lines that had gathered during Roberta's illness and now would stay. Her eyes and heart were full of tears, but she looked straight at him. "No," she said. "You helped my whole family." Rappeport didn't respond, and my mother, biting her lip so she would be able to speak clearly, without crying, made sure he'd understood her. She meant me, as much as Roberta. "My *whole* family," she said again.

It was what I knew she would say, because the truth was there to see. Rappeport never offered a false promise. He is not especially articulate and "not infrequently," as he would say, he puts his foot in it. Despite his high intelligence, he's not as broad-minded as I would like, and sometimes, when his heart slams shut, it hurts. He could do more if he were better able to look beyond his personal disappointments and the constraints that his conventional ideas of status and success place on him. But over and over again, I saw people respond to Rappeport at their most critically important and frightening times, as I did, with love and hope. His seriousness and dedication, the extreme degree of attention he gives to trying to solve the terrible problems of the people in his care, gives them—us—dignity and a sense of purpose.

It is the particularity of his effort that each person consciously feels, but it is its broader scope that supports him and most impacts on them. Though both science and religion teach us that suffering, in both its constant and mutant forms, is here to stay, it is surely morally necessary to try to alleviate and eliminate it each time, and as we can.

Rappeport is right to characterize himself as an activist, a doer. Who would want a doctor who is not? And yet, his most lasting value may be as a conduit. It is he who, as Brian Smith says, carries information from the bedside to the laboratory bench and back again, thus furthering cure. Even more, it is through him that so many people, each with flesh longing to live, and frightened, wondering eyes, and endurance, and bravery for whatever comes, are filtered, and their imprint placed upon us.

I meant to write a book about Rappeport. Through the years I've known him I've been able to close my eyes and see each plane and crease and shadow on his face, and every time I have looked at him, my heart has softened. It sounds as if I am in love, but I have found that the components of my feeling all have names that aren't his: Roberta, first of all. Wesley, and his brother Scott, and his parents Martha and Ed. And now, his wife Kathy. Peter, intelligent and compassionate through all his suffering. Jill Mason. Sis Stott, who died, at fifty-five, of pancreatic cancer in April of 1991— "She never complained," her daughter says. "She was a mother to the last *second*"—and Ricky and both Carls. There are the Houghs: Patrick especially, but Pam and Scott, and Christopher, whom I never knew, and Beverly, who, from the time she was a very little girl, always understood. Beloved Brian Murphy. There are the Frisbees. And Jennie Gossom, full of life and sweetness. Brave, brave Reba, both Ezras, and Daniel. The Schulers, the Thompsons, and Jane. And all the others. Worth saving, through the means of science and medicine, with all the purity of spirit and intelligent inquiry we can find or create.

They are woven together, somehow, in Rappeport, making him a worthy emblem upon the heart.

Notes

INTRODUCTION

1. Conference at Mt. Sinai Hospital, New York, N.Y., November 18, 1989.
2. Ibid.
3. Age limits for bone marrow transplants are, like much about the field, variable and changing. In 1991, forty-five or fifty is a common cutoff point for an allogeneic transplant (the kind a patient with CML would need), but some centers offer them for patients considerably older—though then the risks are correspondingly higher—and alert and progressive doctors continue to reassess the criteria they use in recommending therapy.

CHAPTER 1: *Fundamentals*

1. Most commonly a hematologist, but sometimes an oncologist or immunologist. Hematologists and oncologists often have joint board certification, but usually refer to themselves as one or the other, depending on the emphases of their practices and the hospital division with which they're most closely associated.

Immunologists performed some of the first bone marrow transplants (in the 1960s, on babies suffering from severe combined immunodeficiency). At that time board certification did not exist. Now, although the examination for immunologists is different from that for hematologists/oncologists, the information and expertise necessary for doctors in all three of these specialties is closely allied and overlapping.

2. Rappeport employs this environment for those patients who receive allogeneic transplants—that is, marrow from someone other than themselves. People receiving autologous transplants—that is, getting their own marrow back—receive their treatment in clean, rather than sterile, rooms. The vast majority of Rappeport's patients receive allogeneic, rather than autologous, transplants.

3. Twenty-seven years after Rappeport's early experience, however, bone marrow transplantation has achieved such widespread success that E. Donnall Thomas, who instigated the therapy, first on dogs and then on human beings, and who has persisted and refined it for decades, won the 1990 Nobel Prize in Physiology or Medicine, sharing it with Joseph E. Murray, who was awarded it for his work on kidney transplantation. Gina Kolata, reporting on the award in the October 9, 1990, *New York Times*, quoted the Nobel Committee as saying of both Thomas and Murray that the work they'd accomplished was "crucial for those tens of thousands of severely ill patients who can either be cured or given a decent life when other treatment methods are without success."

4. Doctors vary in the dietary restrictions and in the cleanliness rules they set for patients undergoing bone marrow transplants. Rappeport's rules are conservative.

5. Throughout this book, as throughout academic medicine, doctors at different levels are always present. At the top are attending physicians—doctors, such as Smith and Rappeport, who have completed their formal medical education and training. Next are fellows. They are fully qualified doctors who have already completed several years in a specialty (internal medicine, surgery, pediatrics, or radiology) and are now spending about three years—longer if they do additional research—qualifying for a subspecialty. (Hematology is a subspecialty of internal medicine as, for example, neurosurgery is of surgery or

neonatology of pediatrics.) Lastly, there are house officers, a term that applies to residents and interns. A doctor at the resident level is licensed, and in private practice could work as a general practitioner. As a hospital employee, he or she is training for a specialty. Interns have graduated from medical school and are completing the year of hospital work that will allow them to be licensed.

6. What constitutes an "older" versus a "younger" patient is unclear here, as it is in deciding at what age a person is still young enough to receive a bone marrow transplant. Both questions are subject to ongoing exploration and experimentation.

7. There are a number of genes at the area of chromosome 6 known as the HLA complex. Donor and recipient need not match at all of them for a transplant to be possible.

CHAPTER 2: The Biggest Obstacle

1. James D. Watson, Nancy H. Hopkins, Jeffrey W. Roberts, Joan Argetsinger Steitz, and Alan M. Weiner, *Molecular Biology of the Gene*, vol. 2. (Menlo Park, Cal.: Benjamin/Cummings Publishing Company, Inc., 1987), pp. 1083–84. I am also indebted to Peter Beardsley, chief of pediatric oncology/hematology at Yale University, for his explanation of retinoblastoma.

2. R. E. Billingham, "The Biology of Graft-Versus-Host Reactions," in *The Harvey Lectures 1966–1967* (New York: Academic Press, 1968).

CHAPTER 3: Blood Itself

1. Because cyclosporine prevents graft rejection, it too is useful in transplants for aplastic anemia. And if it does work against GVH, it provides—in aplastic anemia—"a twofer," as Rappeport puts it.

2. Brian Smith says, however, that "some centers do use radiation" in aplastic anemia, "but either at a low dose (designed to be immunosuppressive but not destroy all stem cells) or only directed at the lymphoid tissue (again, so that it acts as an immunosuppressant, but not to kill stem cells)."

3. Lennart Nilsson, *The Body Victorious* (New York: Delacorte, 1987), p. 132.

4. Max F. Perutz, "Should Genes Be Screened?" *The New York Review of Books*, May 18, 1989.

5. Interview with Perutz, Cambridge, England, June 4, 1990. Emended by letter June 6, 1991.

CHAPTER 4: Discovery
1. Robertson Parkman, M.D., Joel Rappeport, M.D., Raif Geha, M.D., James Belli, M.D., Robert Cassady, M.D., Raphael Levey, M.D., David G. Nathan, M.D., and Fred S. Rosen, M.D., "Complete Correction of the Wiskott-Aldrich Syndrome by Allogeneic Bone-Marrow Transplantation," *The New England Journal of Medicine*, April 27, 1978. An earlier attempt, in Wisconsin, at transplanting a child with Wiskott-Aldrich syndrome was a partial success: Fritz H. Bach, M.D., Richard J. Albertini, M.D., James L. Anderson, M.D., Patricia Joo, M.D., Mortimer M. Bortin, M.D., "Bone-Marrow Transplantation in a Patient with the Wiskott-Aldrich Syndrome," *The Lancet*, December 28, 1968. Rappeport says the Wisconsin patient's T cells were normalized, but his platelets remained low.
2. Interview with Rosen, Boston, Mass., March 3, 1990.
3. Parkman, Rappeport et al., "Complete Correction."
4. Rosen interview.
5. Interview with Grosveld, London, June 8, 1990, emended by letter June 17, 1991.
6. Rosen interview.

No notes in CHAPTER 5, "Uncertainty."

CHAPTER 6: Experimentation
1. Interview with Ginns, Bethesda, Md., February 28, 1990.
2. Ibid.
3. Ibid.
4. Joel M. Rappeport, M.D., and Edward I. Ginns, M.D., Ph.D., "Bone-Marrow Transplantation in Severe Gaucher's Disease," *The New England Journal of Medicine*, July 12, 1984.
5. Ginns interview.
6. Ibid.
7. Telephone interview with Barranger, February 15, 1991.
8. Donald B. Kohn, M.D., of Children's Hospital Los Angeles, who made the 1990 report, based it on Olle Ringde, Carl-Gustav Groth, Anders Erikson, Lars Backman, Stappen Granqvist, Jan-Erik Mansson, and Lars Svennerholm, "Long-Term Follow-up of the First Successful Bone Marrow Transplanta-

tion in Gaucher Disease," *Transplantation*, vol. 46, no. 1 (July 1988), pp. 66–70. The Ringde et al. paper also describes the child as mostly "active and healthy 5 years after bone marrow transplantation," and Dr. Kohn adds that because there is no true basis for comparison with this child, the relative rate and significance of her deterioration is difficult to assess.

9. Ginns interview.
10. Rappeport and Ginns, "Bone-Marrow . . . in Gaucher's."
11. Ginns interview.
12. Barranger interview.
13. Ginns interview.
14. Brian Smith says that retrospectively it is clear that the child with hemophilia must have been HIV-positive. Hemophiliacs have normal platelets, he explains, and it is only if the child had had an additional problem—ITP (for immune thrombocytopenic purpura), a disorder that can occur on its own but is sometimes associated with AIDS, and which destroys platelets—that he would have suffered this particular bleeding problem. The clotting component hemophiliacs normally lack is not platelets but Factor VIII, a blood product that is gathered from multiple donors. The tragic result is that before AIDS was identified and the blood supply screened, the vast majority of people with hemophilia were infected with the disease, as a result of their dependency on a blood product pooled from many people.
15. Ginns interview.
16. Barranger interview.
17. Ibid.
18. Rappeport and Ginns, "Bone-Marrow . . . in Gaucher's."
19. Barranger interview.
20. Ibid.

CHAPTER 7: Immunity
1. Joel M. Rappeport, Brian R. Smith, Robertson Parkman, and Fred S. Rosen, "Application of Bone Marrow Transplantation in Genetic Diseases," *Clinics in Haematology*, vol. 12, no. 3 (October 1983), p. 759. The probable reason for this is the young age of the recipients and donors, and the fact that less marrow, with fewer T cells from peripheral blood, is transplanted.
2. Ibid., p. 757.
3. Interview with Rosen, March 3, 1990.

4. Brian R. Smith, John A. Hansen, and Joel M. Rappeport, "Bone Marrow Transplantation: Selecting Donors and Diseases," *Hematology—1991, The Education Program of the American Society of Hematology* (Washington, D.C.: American Society of Hematology, 1991).

5. Rosen interview.

CHAPTER 8: New Prospects

1. MOPP is an acronym for the drugs Mechlorethamine, Oncovin, procarbazine, and prednisone.

2. James M. Jandl, M.D., *Blood: Textbook of Hematology* (Boston: Little, Brown, 1987), p. 871.

3. Rappeport is using the brand name for this drug. Its generic name is cyclophosphamide.

4. Rob Thompson is right to make this stipulation. Despite the terror that intubation causes, many people, including some of Rappeport's very sick patients, are intubated and later—thanks in part to having been intubated when they could not breathe on their own—go on to recover.

5. People who undergo autologous transplants do not need as long a period of near-isolation as do those who have allogeneic transplants because, as Rappeport says, they are immunosuppressed for a shorter time. That is why Jane was able to go to a play six months after her transplant, instead of waiting the year that Rappeport usually imposes on his patients.

CONCLUSION

1. Grosveld interview, June 8, 1990, and letter, June 17, 1991.

2. In making this statement, I am including those people for whom bone marrow transplantation is not an option.

Sources

Most of *Life's Blood* is based on my own observation, and on interviews I conducted between July 1987 and September 1991. In addition, several books and articles were valuable sources of facts and explanation:

Jandl, J. H. *Blood: Textbook of Hematology*. Boston: Little, Brown & Company, 1987.

Mulligan, R. C. "Gene Transfer and Gene Therapy: Principles, Prospects and Perspective." In J. Lindsten and U. Petterson, eds., *Etiology of Human Disease at the DNA Level* (Nobel Symposium 80), chapter 12. New York: Raven Press, 1991.

Nilsson, Lennart. *The Body Victorious*. New York: Delacorte Press, 1985.

Parkman, Robertson; Joel Rappeport; Raif Geha; James Belli; Robert Cassady; Raphael Levey; David G. Nathan; and Fred S. Rosen. "Complete Correction of the Wiskott-Aldrich Syndrome by Allogeneic Bone-Marrow Transplantation." *The New England Journal of Medicine*, April 27, 1978.

Rappeport, Joel M. "Bone Marrow Transplantation." In David G.

Nathan and Frank A. Oski, eds., *Hematology of Infancy and Childhood*. Philadelphia: W. B. Saunders, 1987.

Rappeport, Joel M. "Principles of Bone Marrow Transplantation." In D. E. Peterson, E. G. Elias, and S. T. Sonis, eds., *Head and Neck Management of the Cancer Patient*. The Hague: Martinus Nijhoff Publishing, 1986.

Rappeport, Joel M.; John A. Barranger; and Edward I. Ginns. "Bone Marrow Transplantation in Gaucher Disease." *Birth Defects: Original Article Series*, vol. 22, no. 1, March of Dimes–Birth Defects Foundation, 1986.

Rappeport, Joel M., and Edward I. Ginns. "Bone-Marrow Transplantation in Severe Gaucher's Disease." *The New England Journal of Medicine*, July 12, 1984.

Rappeport, Joel M.; Brian R. Smith; Robertson Parkman; and Fred S. Rosen. "Application of Bone Marrow Transplantation in Genetic Diseases." *Clinics in Haematology*, vol. 12, no. 3 (October 1983).

Smith, Brian R.; John A. Hansen; and Joel M. Rappeport. "Bone Marrow Transplantation: Selecting Donors and Diseases." *Hematology—1991, The Education Program of the American Society of Hematology*. Washington, D.C.: American Society of Hematology, 1991.

Thomas, E. Donnall, M.D. "Bone-Marrow Transplantation." *Cancer Journal for Clinicians*, vol. 37, no. 5 (September/October 1987).

Watson, James D.; Nancy H. Hopkins; Jeffrey W. Roberts; Joan Argetsinger Steitz; and Alan M. Weiner. *Molecular Biology of the Gene*, vols. 1 and 2. Menlo Park, Cal.: Benjamin/Cummings, 1987.

In addition, four books were wonderful philosophical and literary examples and teachers, helping me to think and write about people:

Dorris, M. *The Broken Cord*. New York: Harper & Row, 1989.

Murdoch, Iris. *The Sovereignty of Good*. New York: Routledge & Kegan Paul, 1986.

Sontag, Susan. *Illness as Metaphor*. New York: Vintage Books, 1979.

Wilkes, Paul. *In Mysterious Ways*. New York: Random House, 1990.

Acknowledgments

Brian Smith helped me at every stage, and in every way, with this book. He made valuable suggestions, gave detailed explanations of medicine and science, answered countless questions, and gave multiple painstaking readings of the manuscript. He also offered perceptive and sympathetic advice and insight about the people and issues that concerned me in my research and writing. Most important, his good humor and the constancy of his kind friendship supported me during hard times and, always, enlivened my task.

The dignity, openness, and grace with which patients and their families showed me their bravery and told me of their suffering was a spiritual and intellectual education. My debt to everyone named in the text is enormous. I thank also the people whose stories I haven't included, though they helped inform me, especially Khaled Al Hegelan, Kathy Gillette Anderson, Christine Berl, Daniel Berl, Martha Berl, Richard Berl, Cheryl Charpentier, Lorraine Cohen, Don and Debbie Dragon, Jay and June Halloran, Joseph Montuori, Josephine and Patrick Montuori, Sr., Patrick Montuori, Jr., Miranda Russell and Bill Crozier, and Jeffrey Shinn. Nancy Potter's will to do good is matched only by her humility. I add my thanks for the example she gives, and for her kindness, to those of everyone who knows her.

In addition to those doctors and scientists I describe and quote in the book, many others gave background and new information, particularly Dr. James Armitage, Chairman of the Department of Internal Medicine, University of Nebraska; Dr. Edward Benz, Chief, Section of Hematology, and Professor of Internal Medicine and Genetics at the Yale University School of Medicine; Dr. Ernest Beutler, Chairman, Department of Molecular and Experimental Medicine, Scripps Clinic and Research Foundation; Professor E. C. Gordon-Smith, Department of Cellular and Molecular Sciences, Division of Haematology, St. George's Hospital Medical School; Professor Kenneth K. Kidd, Department of Genetics, Yale University School of Medicine; Professor David Linch, Department of Haematology, University College and Middlesex School of Medicine; Dr. Richard O'Reilly, Chairman of the Department of Pediatrics and Chief of the Bone Marrow Transplantation Service, Memorial Sloan-Kettering Cancer Center; Dr. Robertson Parkman, Head, Division of Research Immunology and Bone Marrow Transplantation, Children's Hospital, Los Angeles; Professor Frank H. Ruddle, Chairman of the Department of Biology, Yale University; Dr. Cynthia Rutherford, Director of the Donor and Transfusion Service, Brigham and Women's Hospital; Dr. Nancy Tarbell, Division Chief of Radiation Oncology, Children's Hospital, Boston; and Professor Sir David Weatherall, FRS, Nuffield Department of Clinical Medicine, John Radcliffe Hospital, University of Oxford.

I am grateful to Dr. Louis Wasserman, Distinguished Service Professor Emeritus, Mt. Sinai School of Medicine, for showing me the happiness which his energetic, intelligent, and useful life in hematology has brought him, and to Dr. Eugene Cronkite, Emeritus Chairman and Senior Scientist, Medical Department, Brookhaven National Laboratory, for sharing with me not only some of his knowledge but also his phenomenal energy and integrity.

Professor Phillip A. Sharp, Head of the Department of Biology at the Massachusetts Institute of Technology, gave a careful reading of the manuscript and excellent advice. Dr. Dorothy J. Ganick, pediatric hematologist/oncologist, Webster Clinic, Green Bay and Children's Hospital of Wisconsin, checked the first draft, chapter by chapter, for accuracy and offered encouragement and criticism from the beginning and straight through. David M.

Kennedy and Philip P. Hallie, Professor Emeritus of Philosophy and the Humanities at Wesleyan University, both read the first half of the manuscript at an early stage and gave generous, thoughtful assessments.

For readings and other favors and kindnesses, often over many years, I am grateful also to Alan Brewster, Robert Brown, Ellen Epstein, Irving Epstein, Milly Glimcher, Nancy Kruger, Susan Lang, Susan Michaelson, Donna Umana Newcomb, Jeanne O'Reilly, Judy Rinard, Suzanne Schneider, John Schnittker, Pamela Reed Shufro, Steven Shufro, and Susan Werbe. My dear friend Joan Davidson gave, as always, hospitality, interest, and support. Dr. Simon Kroll and Mary Kroll welcomed me to England, offered information, and gave friendship. Thanks also to William and Lucy Kroll.

Peter Steinfels and Margaret O'Brien Steinfels have given me opportunity, as well as their interest and encouragement. Both Peter and Peggy read the first part of the manuscript and offered suggestions. I am especially grateful to Peggy for recommending Iris Murdoch's work to me, and to Peter for submitting the sample that became *Life's Blood* to Simon & Schuster.

At Simon & Schuster, George Hodgman has shown intelligence and compassion from the beginning and has been companion and sensitive critic, as well as editor and advocate, in my enterprise. Thanks also to Carole Lalli, for generous guidance early on. Felice Einhorn and Emily Remes offered counsel that was both sympathetic and authoritative. Toni Rachiele's caring punctiliousness was a reassuring challenge. Alice Mayhew told me to "write up to the reader," and thus gave me the most inspiring advice I have ever received.

Helen Rees, my agent, has been diplomatic, efficient, and kind. Her succinct insights stay with me.

I am grateful to Doris Marget Pinsley, my mother, for the mixture of enthusiasm and wisdom she gave me throughout the writing of this book. My debt to my sister Roberta is incalculable and profound. Allen Schultz, Roberta's husband, has been unfailing in his loving support, as have Roberta and Allen's children: Emily, Edward, James, and Andrew, who also, with their gentle understanding, gave me peace of mind.

My husband Ernie Zupancic is the critical central example of goodness in my life. He has given me every kind of help, present in various visible and invisible ways, on every page.

My greatest thanks go to my children: Meg, Charlie, and Nellie Zupancic. Each of them gave involvement, kindness, and intelligence, often beyond their years. Most of all, the tenderness and joy they convey reminds me, always, of the value and beauty of life.

Index